Food, Mood & Health Journal
The Happiness Project:
Plan Your Way Back to Health
in 120 Days

Ladbroke Grove Press

Disclaimer:

The publisher has put forth its best efforts in preparing and formatting this book. The information provided within by our author is provided 'as is' and you read and use this information at your own risk. The publisher is not a medical professional. And you should consult your doctor before engaging in any new or strenuous activities. The publisher and author disclaim any liabilities for any loss of profit, commercial or personal damages resulting from the use of information contained in this book.

Your suggestions/comments are always welcome.
Ladbroke Grove Press

www.ladbrokegrovepress.com
contact@ladbrokegrovepress.com

Everyone wants to be healthy, but very few of us take action to make this happen.

Congratulations! Small steps make big changes, and in this convenient, discreet, purse sized journal, you can track your moods, eating habits, and exercise goals for the next 120 days. Plus now including 25 bonus Daily Planners to ensure your new healthy behaviors become a habit!

There is no need to stare at a blank page and wonder what to write. Follow the guides on each page, check in with your moods, eating habits, portion control, snacks, exercise, and this ultimate **Food, Mood & Health Journal** will be your companion as you retrain your brain and body to learn positive new habits, as you improve your physical and mental wellbeing.

And at the completion of this journal, you will be well on your way to a healthier, happier you. Let's get started.

Tips for Using Your Food, Mood & Health Journal:

*Did you know that studies show that individuals who keep a food journal and record their eating wellness and fitness goals lose twice as much weight as those who don't?

*Actually use the journal. It looks great in your purse or glove compartment, but even better in in your hand, with a pen in the other.

*Actually review your entries. Schedule a weekly review of your past entries. Do you notice any trends, days or meals where you were stuck? All of this information is gold.

*Know WHY you want to journal your food intake/patterns, moods and exercise.

*It is all about building AWARENESS of what and why you are eating. Mindfulness is what we are striving for, really paying attention to what and why we are eating. Are you really hungry or is it stress?

Daily Planner (example)

Date: _May 3, 2015_ Weight: _138 POUNDS_

- **What did you eat and How much did you eat?**
- **How was it prepared? (Ex: Homemade, fast food)**
- **Where did you get your food? (Ex: At home, cafe)**
- **Where did you eat? (Ex: At home, cafe, in car)**
- **Who did you eat with? (Ex: By myself, with family)**

BREAKFAST:
INSTANT OATMEAL (1 PACKET), ALMOND MILK (1/2 CUP,

2 TEASPOONS CHOPPED WALNUTS, 1 HARD BOILED EGG,
TEA (1 CUP, NO SWEETENER)

SNACK:
1 MEDIUM PINK LADY APPLE, 1 LOW FAT STRING CHEESE, 1

BOTTLE FILTERED WATER (LG- 16 OZ)

LUNCH:
TACO SALAD (MIXED LETTUCE, CARROT, AVOCADO CUBES,) +

SEASONED TOFU CUBES (1/2 CUP), 1 TB LOW FAT SOUR
CREAM + WATER MINERAL, 1 GLASS

SNACK: HANDFUL OF UNSALTED ALMONDS, 1 STEVIA
SWEETENED

SODA (12 OZ)

DINNER: + 2 GLASSES WATER (FILTERED)
SALMON (BAKED WITH LEMON JUICE + DILL) FIST SIZED

PORTION, STEAMED ASPARAGUS (8 SPEARS), 1/2 CUP
QUINOA.

SNACK: LOW FAT PLAIN GREEK YOGURT (8 OZ) WITH
HANDFUL
OF BLUEBERRIES ON TOP, DECAF BLACK TEA (1 CUP)

Keepin' Hydrated! 8 x 8 oz. of water each day.

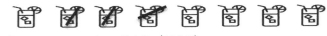

+ 2 TEA, GREEN AND BLACK (DECAF)

Exercise Today (Time & Type)
YOGA, 30 MINS, CORE FOCUS. MEDITATION 10 MINS X 2.

What's Your Mood: Happy, quiet, sad, hopeful, bored, exhausted, lonely, peaceful, tired, stressed, joyful, calm?   Make a note:

TIRED, DEADLINES- STRESSED, HAPPY I ATE WELL TODAY

What's My Day Been Like? Any Triggers? (Times, People, Moods, Situations)

BUSY, LOTS OF PEOPLE NEEDING MY ATTENTION, LOW MOOD IN EVENING, GLAD TO RELAX WITH FINAL SNACK.

What I Will Pay More Attention To: (Behaviors/Actions)

SLOW DOWN AND PAY ATTENTION TO WHAT I AM EATING ESP. MY SNACKS!! MORE H2O IN THE MORNING.

How Did I Do Today?
☐ Brilliant   x Really Well   ☐ Just Okay
☐ I'll Focus On Doing Better Tomorrow

What Does Your Average Plate Look Like?

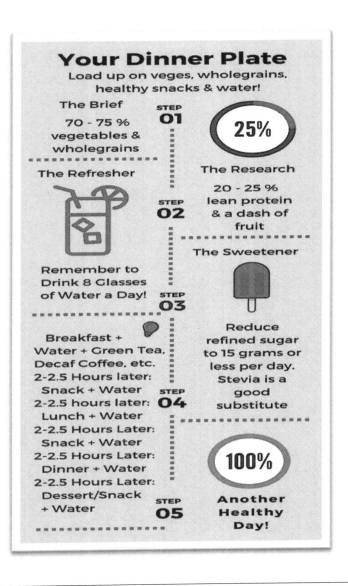

Your Dinner Plate

Load up on veges, wholegrains, healthy snacks & water!

The Brief

70 - 75 % vegetables & wholegrains

STEP 01

25%

The Refresher

STEP 02

The Research

20 - 25 % lean protein & a dash of fruit

Remember to Drink 8 Glasses of Water a Day!

STEP 03

The Sweetener

Breakfast + Water + Green Tea, Decaf Coffee, etc. 2-2.5 Hours later: Snack + Water 2-2.5 hours later: Lunch + Water 2-2.5 Hours Later: Snack + Water 2-2.5 Hours Later: Dinner + Water 2-2.5 Hours Later: Dessert/Snack + Water

STEP 04

Reduce refined sugar to 15 grams or less per day. Stevia is a good substitute

STEP 05

100%

Another Healthy Day!

Did You Know It's Good to Have Snacks!

- Maintains consistent blood sugar levels.
- Ensures you don't feel deprived.
- Busy people need consistent fuel.
- Keep energy levels high.
- Healthy fats are necessary, bad ones are not!
- But the snacks must be healthy (low fat, plenty of vegetables).
- For example:

Creamy white bean dip and vege sticks, garlicky homemade hummus & pita chips (Recipes can be found in: The DASH Diet Low Salt Recipes Book)

But Sugar is a No No

- Try not to have more than 15 grams of refined sugar a day.
- Stevia is delicious, natural and available in drops to flavor mineral water (cola is yummy), granulated for baking, cereal and drinks.

My Goals and Inspiration

At the end of each day, take time to look at your planner entries and write a few sentences to reflect on what your meal choices were and your goals for tomorrow.

Remember to celebrate the victories, no matter how small they are!

- How often did you think of your health and nutrition when making food choices? What were some of your healthiest choices?
- Were any of your food choices influenced by ads on TV or in magazines?
- How many times today did you eat because you were actually hungry?
- Was today a typical day for you? Were there any other factors that affected what you ate today?

Daily Planner

Date: 6|20|2016 Weight:

Meals	What & How Much?	How was it prepared?	Where did you get your food?	Where did you eat?	Who did you eat with?

Breakfast – Home
- 4 medium sized pancakes
- 16 oz. caramel coffee w/ creamer

Snack – Office
- small bag dill pickle potato chips
- 22 oz. Dr. Pepper $2.06

Lunch

Snack

5 oreos

Dinner

alfredo

3 pieces of garlic bread

1 glass of wine

**Dessert/
Snack**

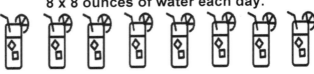

Keepin' Hydrated!
8 x 8 ounces of water each day.

Exercise Today (Time & Type of Workouts)

walk around block

steps: 5076

What's Your Mood: Happy, quiet, sad, hopeful, bored, exhausted, lonely, peaceful, tired, stressed, joyful, calm?   Make a note:

stressed: Research paper, hours, stomach troubles

What's My Day Been Like? Any Triggers? (Times, People, Moods, Situations)

- stressful morning
- headache around 4:15

What I Will Pay More Attention To: (Behaviors/Actions)

- taking meds on time
- not wasting time

How Did I Do Today?

☐ Brilliant   ☐ Really Well ☐ Just Okay
☒ I'll Focus On Doing Better Tomorrow

"Every accomplishment starts with the willingness to try."

Daily Planner

Date: 6/21/2016   Weight:

Meals	What & How Much?	How was it prepared?	Where did you get your food?	Where did you eat?	Who did you eat with?

Breakfast
- bowl of lucky charms
- 8 oz. caramel coffee w/ creamer

Snack
- black cherry Greek yogurt
- doughnut
- orange juice

Lunch
- small order pretzel bites
- large frappuccino

$10.06

Snack

- blackberries

Dinner

- salad w/ ranch
- ½ bottle of Pepsi

**Dessert/
Snack**

- frosted brownie

Keepin' Hydrated!
8 x 8 ounces of water each day.

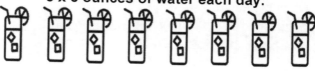

Exercise Today (Time & Type of Workouts)

_____ STEPS: 5233

What's Your Mood: Happy, quiet, sad, hopeful, bored, exhausted, lonely, peaceful, tired, stressed, joyful, calm? **Make a note:**

What's My Day Been Like? Any Triggers? (Times, People, Moods, Situations)

What I Will Pay More Attention To: (Behaviors/Actions)

• try to take stairs more

How Did I Do Today?

☐ **Brilliant** ☐ **Really Well** ☐ **Just Okay**
☒ **I'll Focus On Doing Better Tomorrow**

"Just take it a day at a time."

Daily Planner

Date: 6/22/2016 Weight:

Meals	What & How Much?	How was it prepared?	Where did you get your food?	Where did you eat?	Who did you eat with?

Breakfast

- brownie
- cheese omelet
- 1 piece buttered toast

Snack

- large iced chai latte

$4.58

Lunch

- chipotle veggie burrito
- inta juice smoothie

Snack

Dinner

**Dessert/
Snack**

Keepin' Hydrated!
8 x 8 ounces of water each day.

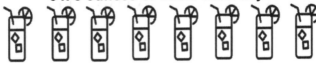

Exercise Today (Time & Type of Workouts)

STEPS: **5673**

What's Your Mood: Happy, quiet, sad, hopeful, bored, exhausted, lonely, peaceful, tired, stressed, joyful, calm? Make a note:

What's My Day Been Like? Any Triggers? (Times, People, Moods, Situations)

What I Will Pay More Attention To: (Behaviors/Actions)

• take stairs

How Did I Do Today?

☐ **Brilliant** ☐ **Really Well** ☐ **Just Okay**
☐ **I'll Focus On Doing Better Tomorrow**

"Small steps equal big changes."

Daily Planner

Date: 6|23|2016   Weight:

Meals	What & How Much?	How was it prepared?	Where did you get your food?	Where did you eat?	Who did you eat with?

Breakfast
- brownie
- chocolate malt
- 1 piece buttered toast
- couple bites of cheese omelet

Snack
- dry cereal - Berries

Lunch
- mac 'n' cheese
- apple

Snack

- baked cheetos
- 1 piece dark chocolate

Dinner

- cheese curds
- Dirty Shirley

Dessert/ Snack

- "cast iron cookie" & ice cream

Keepin' Hydrated!
8 x 8 ounces of water each day.

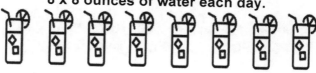

Exercise Today (Time & Type of Workouts)

What's Your Mood: Happy, quiet, sad, hopeful, bored, exhausted, lonely, peaceful, tired, stressed, joyful, calm?   **Make a note:**

What's My Day Been Like? Any Triggers? (Times, People, Moods, Situations)

What I Will Pay More Attention To: (Behaviors/Actions)

How Did I Do Today?

☐ **Brilliant**   ☐ **Really Well** ☐ **Just Okay**
☐ **I'll Focus On Doing Better Tomorrow**

"Every accomplishment starts with the willingness to try."

Daily Planner

Date: 6/24/2016 Weight:

Meals	What & How Much?	How was it prepared?	Where did you get your food?	Where did you eat?	Who did you eat with?

Breakfast

- Cereal — Honey comb
- Vanilla Frappuccino

Snack

- cinnamon crunch bagel w/ honey walnut cream cheese
- pretzels

Lunch

Snack

Dinner

**Dessert/
Snack**

Keepin' Hydrated!
8 x 8 ounces of water each day.

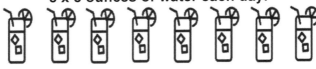

Exercise Today (Time & Type of Workouts)

What's Your Mood: Happy, quiet, sad, hopeful, bored, exhausted, lonely, peaceful, tired, stressed, joyful, calm?   **Make a note:**

What's My Day Been Like? Any Triggers? (Times, People, Moods, Situations)

What I Will Pay More Attention To: (Behaviors/Actions)

How Did I Do Today?

☐ **Brilliant**   ☐ **Really Well** ☐ **Just Okay**
☐ **I'll Focus On Doing Better Tomorrow**

"Every change can be met with your determination."

Daily Planner

Date: _____ Weight: _____

Meals	What & How Much?	How was it prepared?	Where did you get your food?	Where did you eat?	Who did you eat with?
Breakfast					
Snack					
Lunch					

Snack

Dinner

**Dessert/
Snack**

Keepin' Hydrated!
8 x 8 ounces of water each day.

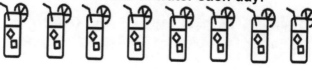

Exercise Today (Time & Type of Workouts)

What's Your Mood: Happy, quiet, sad, hopeful, bored, exhausted, lonely, peaceful, tired, stressed, joyful, calm?   **Make a note:**

What's My Day Been Like? Any Triggers? (Times, People, Moods, Situations)

What I Will Pay More Attention To: (Behaviors/Actions)

How Did I Do Today?

☐ **Brilliant**   ☐ **Really Well** ☐ **Just Okay**
☐ **I'll Focus On Doing Better Tomorrow**

"Change is uncomfortable at first, but soon it becomes habit."

Daily Planner

Date: Weight:

Meals	What & How Much?	How was it prepared?	Where did you get your food?	Where did you eat?	Who did you eat with?
Breakfast					
Snack					
Lunch					

Snack

Dinner

**Dessert/
Snack**

Keepin' Hydrated!
8 x 8 ounces of water each day.

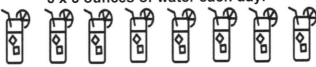

Exercise Today (Time & Type of Workouts)

What's Your Mood: Happy, quiet, sad, hopeful, bored, exhausted, lonely, peaceful, tired, stressed, joyful, calm? **Make a note:**

What's My Day Been Like? Any Triggers? (Times, People, Moods, Situations)

What I Will Pay More Attention To: (Behaviors/Actions)

How Did I Do Today?

☐ **Brilliant**   ☐ **Really Well** ☐ **Just Okay**
☐ **I'll Focus On Doing Better Tomorrow**

"Every accomplishment starts with the willingness to try."

Daily Planner

Date: _____ Weight: _____

Meals	What & How Much?	How was it prepared?	Where did you get your food?	Where did you eat?	Who did you eat with?
Breakfast					
Snack					
Lunch					

Snack

Dinner

**Dessert/
Snack**

Keepin' Hydrated!
8 x 8 ounces of water each day.

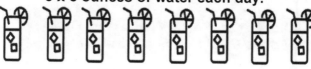

Exercise Today (Time & Type of Workouts)

What's Your Mood: Happy, quiet, sad, hopeful, bored, exhausted, lonely, peaceful, tired, stressed, joyful, calm?   **Make a note:**

What's My Day Been Like? Any Triggers? (Times, People, Moods, Situations)

What I Will Pay More Attention To: (Behaviors/Actions)

How Did I Do Today?

☐ **Brilliant**   ☐ **Really Well** ☐ **Just Okay**
☐ **I'll Focus On Doing Better Tomorrow**

"Take it a day at a time."

Daily Planner

Date: Weight:

Meals	What & How Much?	How was it prepared?	Where did you get your food?	Where did you eat?	Who did you eat with?
Breakfast					
Snack					
Lunch					

Snack

Dinner

**Dessert/
Snack**

Keepin' Hydrated!
8 x 8 ounces of water each day.

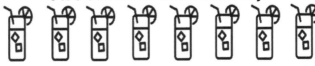

Exercise Today (Time & Type of Workouts)

What's Your Mood: Happy, quiet, sad, hopeful, bored, exhausted, lonely, peaceful, tired, stressed, joyful, calm?   **Make a note:**

What's My Day Been Like? Any Triggers? (Times, People, Moods, Situations)

What I Will Pay More Attention To: (Behaviors/Actions)

How Did I Do Today?

□ **Brilliant**   □ **Really Well** □ **Just Okay**
□ **I'll Focus On Doing Better Tomorrow**

"You've got this!"

Daily Planner

Date: Weight:

Meals	What & How Much?	How was it prepared?	Where did you get your food?	Where did you eat?	Who did you eat with?
Breakfast					
Snack					
Lunch					

Snack

Dinner

**Dessert/
Snack**

Keepin' Hydrated!
8 x 8 ounces of water each day.

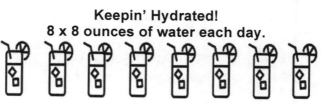

Exercise Today (Time & Type of Workouts)

What's Your Mood: Happy, quiet, sad, hopeful, bored, exhausted, lonely, peaceful, tired, stressed, joyful, calm?   **Make a note:**

What's My Day Been Like? Any Triggers? (Times, People, Moods, Situations)

What I Will Pay More Attention To: (Behaviors/Actions)

How Did I Do Today?

☐ **Brilliant**   ☐ **Really Well** ☐ **Just Okay**
☐ **I'll Focus On Doing Better Tomorrow**

"Small steps equal big changes."

Daily Planner

Date: Weight:

Meals	What & How Much?	How was it prepared?	Where did you get your food?	Where did you eat?	Who did you eat with?
Breakfast					
Snack					
Lunch					

Snack

Dinner

**Dessert/
Snack**

Keepin' Hydrated!
8 x 8 ounces of water each day.

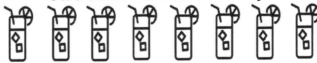

Exercise Today (Time & Type of Workouts)

What's Your Mood: Happy, quiet, sad, hopeful, bored, exhausted, lonely, peaceful, tired, stressed, joyful, calm?   **Make a note:**

What's My Day Been Like? Any Triggers? (Times, People, Moods, Situations)

What I Will Pay More Attention To: (Behaviors/Actions)

How Did I Do Today?

☐ **Brilliant**   ☐ **Really Well** ☐ **Just Okay**
☐ **I'll Focus On Doing Better Tomorrow**

"Accept that you will be successful."

Daily Planner

Date: Weight:

Meals	What & How Much?	How was it prepared?	Where did you get your food?	Where did you eat?	Who did you eat with?
Breakfast					
Snack					
Lunch					

Snack

Dinner

**Dessert/
Snack**

Keepin' Hydrated!
8 x 8 ounces of water each day.

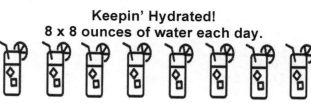

Exercise Today (Time & Type of Workouts)

What's Your Mood: Happy, quiet, sad, hopeful, bored, exhausted, lonely, peaceful, tired, stressed, joyful, calm? **Make a note:**

What's My Day Been Like? Any Triggers? (Times, People, Moods, Situations)

What I Will Pay More Attention To: (Behaviors/Actions)

How Did I Do Today?

☐ **Brilliant**   ☐ **Really Well** ☐ **Just Okay**
☐ **I'll Focus On Doing Better Tomorrow**

"Every accomplishment starts with the willingness to try."

Daily Planner

Date: Weight:

Meals	What & How Much?	How was it prepared?	Where did you get your food?	Where did you eat?	Who did you eat with?
Breakfast					
Snack					
Lunch					

Snack

Dinner

**Dessert/
Snack**

Keepin' Hydrated!
8 x 8 ounces of water each day.

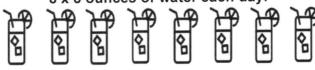

Exercise Today (Time & Type of Workouts)

What's Your Mood: Happy, quiet, sad, hopeful, bored, exhausted, lonely, peaceful, tired, stressed, joyful, calm?　　　**Make a note:**

What's My Day Been Like? Any Triggers? (Times, People, Moods, Situations)

What I Will Pay More Attention To: (Behaviors/Actions)

How Did I Do Today?

☐ **Brilliant**　　☐ **Really Well** ☐ **Just Okay**
☐ **I'll Focus On Doing Better Tomorrow**

"Expect and accept all that is good around you."

Daily Planner

Date: _____   Weight: _____

Meals	What & How Much?	How was it prepared?	Where did you get your food?	Where did you eat?	Who did you eat with?
Breakfast					
Snack					
Lunch					

Snack

Dinner

**Dessert/
Snack**

Keepin' Hydrated!
8 x 8 ounces of water each day.

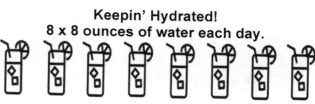

Exercise Today (Time & Type of Workouts)

What's Your Mood: Happy, quiet, sad, hopeful, bored, exhausted, lonely, peaceful, tired, stressed, joyful, calm?   **Make a note:**

What's My Day Been Like? Any Triggers? (Times, People, Moods, Situations)

What I Will Pay More Attention To: (Behaviors/Actions)

How Did I Do Today?

☐ **Brilliant**   ☐ **Really Well** ☐ **Just Okay**
☐ **I'll Focus On Doing Better Tomorrow**

"Every accomplishment starts with the willingness to try."

Daily Planner

Date: Weight:

Meals	What & How Much?	How was it prepared?	Where did you get your food?	Where did you eat?	Who did you eat with?
Breakfast					
Snack					
Lunch					

Snack

Dinner

**Dessert/
Snack**

Keepin' Hydrated!
8 x 8 ounces of water each day.

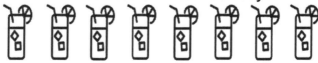

Exercise Today (Time & Type of Workouts)

What's Your Mood: Happy, quiet, sad, hopeful, bored, exhausted, lonely, peaceful, tired, stressed, joyful, calm? **Make a note:**

What's My Day Been Like? Any Triggers? (Times, People, Moods, Situations)

What I Will Pay More Attention To: (Behaviors/Actions)

How Did I Do Today?

☐ **Brilliant** ☐ **Really Well** ☐ **Just Okay**
☐ **I'll Focus On Doing Better Tomorrow**

"You've got this."

Daily Planner

Date: _____ Weight: _____

Meals	What & How Much?	How was it prepared?	Where did you get your food?	Where did you eat?	Who did you eat with?
Breakfast					
Snack					
Lunch					

Snack

Dinner

**Dessert/
Snack**

Keepin' Hydrated!
8 x 8 ounces of water each day.

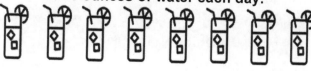

Exercise Today (Time & Type of Workouts)

What's Your Mood: Happy, quiet, sad, hopeful, bored, exhausted, lonely, peaceful, tired, stressed, joyful, calm?   **Make a note:**

What's My Day Been Like? Any Triggers? (Times, People, Moods, Situations)

What I Will Pay More Attention To: (Behaviors/Actions)

How Did I Do Today?

☐ **Brilliant**   ☐ **Really Well** ☐ **Just Okay**
☐ **I'll Focus On Doing Better Tomorrow**

"Every accomplishment starts with the willingness to try."

Daily Planner

Date: _____   Weight: _____

Meals	What & How Much?	How was it prepared?	Where did you get your food?	Where did you eat?	Who did you eat with?
Breakfast					
Snack					
Lunch					

Snack

Dinner

**Dessert/
Snack**

Keepin' Hydrated!
8 x 8 ounces of water each day.

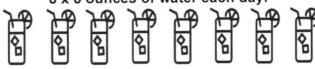

Exercise Today (Time & Type of Workouts)

What's Your Mood: Happy, quiet, sad, hopeful, bored, exhausted, lonely, peaceful, tired, stressed, joyful, calm?   **Make a note:**

What's My Day Been Like? Any Triggers? (Times, People, Moods, Situations)

What I Will Pay More Attention To: (Behaviors/Actions)

How Did I Do Today?

☐ **Brilliant**   ☐ **Really Well** ☐ **Just Okay**
☐ **I'll Focus On Doing Better Tomorrow**

"Every new day is a chance to begin again."

Daily Planner

Date: Weight:

Meals	What & How Much?	How was it prepared?	Where did you get your food?	Where did you eat?	Who did you eat with?
Breakfast					
Snack					
Lunch					

Snack

Dinner

**Dessert/
Snack**

Keepin' Hydrated!
8 x 8 ounces of water each day.

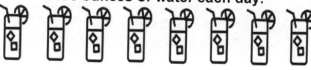

Exercise Today (Time & Type of Workouts)

What's Your Mood: Happy, quiet, sad, hopeful, bored, exhausted, lonely, peaceful, tired, stressed, joyful, calm? Make a note:

What's My Day Been Like? Any Triggers? (Times, People, Moods, Situations)

What I Will Pay More Attention To: (Behaviors/Actions)

How Did I Do Today?

☐ **Brilliant** ☐ **Really Well** ☐ **Just Okay**
☐ **I'll Focus On Doing Better Tomorrow**

"You are more special than you know."

Daily Planner

Date: Weight:

Meals	What & How Much?	How was it prepared?	Where did you get your food?	Where did you eat?	Who did you eat with?
Breakfast					
Snack					
Lunch					

Snack

Dinner

**Dessert/
Snack**

Keepin' Hydrated!
8 x 8 ounces of water each day.

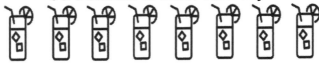

Exercise Today (Time & Type of Workouts)

What's Your Mood: Happy, quiet, sad, hopeful, bored, exhausted, lonely, peaceful, tired, stressed, joyful, calm?   **Make a note:**

What's My Day Been Like? Any Triggers?
(Times, People, Moods, Situations)

What I Will Pay More Attention To:
(Behaviors/Actions)

How Did I Do Today?

☐ **Brilliant**   ☐ **Really Well** ☐ **Just Okay**
☐ **I'll Focus On Doing Better Tomorrow**

"Take it a day at a time."

Daily Planner

Date: Weight:

Meals	What & How Much?	How was it prepared?	Where did you get your food?	Where did you eat?	Who did you eat with?
Breakfast					
Snack					
Lunch					

Snack

Dinner

**Dessert/
Snack**

Keepin' Hydrated!
8 x 8 ounces of water each day.

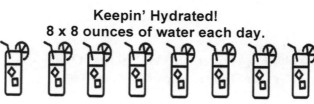

Exercise Today (Time & Type of Workouts)

What's Your Mood: Happy, quiet, sad, hopeful, bored, exhausted, lonely, peaceful, tired, stressed, joyful, calm?   **Make a note:**

What's My Day Been Like? Any Triggers? (Times, People, Moods, Situations)

What I Will Pay More Attention To: (Behaviors/Actions)

How Did I Do Today?

☐ **Brilliant**   ☐ **Really Well** ☐ **Just Okay**
☐ **I'll Focus On Doing Better Tomorrow**

"Pay attention to your thoughts. Are they kind ones?"

Daily Planner

Date: Weight:

Meals	What & How Much?	How was it prepared?	Where did you get your food?	Where did you eat?	Who did you eat with?
Breakfast					
Snack					
Lunch					

Snack

Dinner

**Dessert/
Snack**

Keepin' Hydrated!
8 x 8 ounces of water each day.

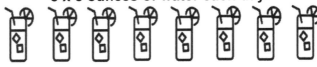

Exercise Today (Time & Type of Workouts)

What's Your Mood: Happy, quiet, sad, hopeful, bored, exhausted, lonely, peaceful, tired, stressed, joyful, calm?   **Make a note:**

What's My Day Been Like? Any Triggers? (Times, People, Moods, Situations)

What I Will Pay More Attention To: (Behaviors/Actions)

How Did I Do Today?

☐ **Brilliant**   ☐ **Really Well** ☐ **Just Okay**
☐ **I'll Focus On Doing Better Tomorrow**

"Every accomplishment starts with the willingness to try."

Daily Planner

Date: Weight:

Meals	What & How Much?	How was it prepared?	Where did you get your food?	Where did you eat?	Who did you eat with?
Breakfast					
Snack					
Lunch					

Snack

Dinner

**Dessert/
Snack**

Keepin' Hydrated!
8 x 8 ounces of water each day.

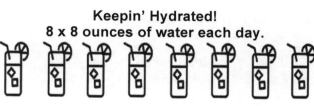

Exercise Today (Time & Type of Workouts)

What's Your Mood: Happy, quiet, sad, hopeful, bored, exhausted, lonely, peaceful, tired, stressed, joyful, calm?   **Make a note:**

What's My Day Been Like? Any Triggers? (Times, People, Moods, Situations)

What I Will Pay More Attention To: (Behaviors/Actions)

How Did I Do Today?

☐ **Brilliant**   ☐ **Really Well** ☐ **Just Okay**
☐ **I'll Focus On Doing Better Tomorrow**

"Look in the mirror and see a miracle, because you are."

Daily Planner

Date: Weight:

Meals	What & How Much?	How was it prepared?	Where did you get your food?	Where did you eat?	Who did you eat with?
Breakfast					
Snack					
Lunch					

Snack

Dinner

**Dessert/
Snack**

Keepin' Hydrated!
8 x 8 ounces of water each day.

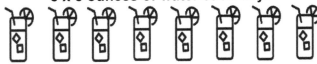

Exercise Today (Time & Type of Workouts)

What's Your Mood: Happy, quiet, sad, hopeful, bored, exhausted, lonely, peaceful, tired, stressed, joyful, calm?   **Make a note:**

What's My Day Been Like? Any Triggers? (Times, People, Moods, Situations)

What I Will Pay More Attention To: (Behaviors/Actions)

How Did I Do Today?

☐ **Brilliant**   ☐ **Really Well** ☐ **Just Okay**
☐ **I'll Focus On Doing Better Tomorrow**

"Every accomplishment starts with the willingness to try."

Daily Planner

Date: Weight:

Meals	What & How Much?	How was it prepared?	Where did you get your food?	Where did you eat?	Who did you eat with?
Breakfast					
Snack					
Lunch					

Snack

Dinner

**Dessert/
Snack**

Keepin' Hydrated!
8 x 8 ounces of water each day.

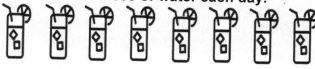

Exercise Today (Time & Type of Workouts)

What's Your Mood: Happy, quiet, sad, hopeful, bored, exhausted, lonely, peaceful, tired, stressed, joyful, calm?   **Make a note:**

What's My Day Been Like? Any Triggers? (Times, People, Moods, Situations)

What I Will Pay More Attention To: (Behaviors/Actions)

How Did I Do Today?

☐ **Brilliant**   ☐ **Really Well** ☐ **Just Okay**
☐ **I'll Focus On Doing Better Tomorrow**

"Expect and accept that you are going to be successful."

Daily Planner

Date: Weight:

Meals	What & How Much?	How was it prepared?	Where did you get your food?	Where did you eat?	Who did you eat with?
Breakfast					
Snack					
Lunch					

Snack

Dinner

**Dessert/
Snack**

Keepin' Hydrated!
8 x 8 ounces of water each day.

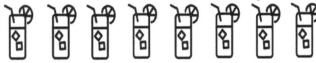

Exercise Today (Time & Type of Workouts)

What's Your Mood: Happy, quiet, sad, hopeful, bored, exhausted, lonely, peaceful, tired, stressed, joyful, calm? **Make a note:**

What's My Day Been Like? Any Triggers? (Times, People, Moods, Situations)

What I Will Pay More Attention To: (Behaviors/Actions)

How Did I Do Today?

☐ **Brilliant** ☐ **Really Well** ☐ **Just Okay**
☐ **I'll Focus On Doing Better Tomorrow**

"The world is a better place with you in it."

Daily Planner

Date: Weight:

Meals	What & How Much?	How was it prepared?	Where did you get your food?	Where did you eat?	Who did you eat with?
Breakfast					
Snack					
Lunch					

Snack

Dinner

**Dessert/
Snack**

Keepin' Hydrated!
8 x 8 ounces of water each day.

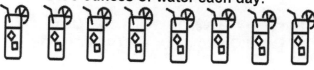

Exercise Today (Time & Type of Workouts)

What's Your Mood: Happy, quiet, sad, hopeful, bored, exhausted, lonely, peaceful, tired, stressed, joyful, calm?   **Make a note:**

What's My Day Been Like? Any Triggers? (Times, People, Moods, Situations)

What I Will Pay More Attention To: (Behaviors/Actions)

How Did I Do Today?

□ **Brilliant**   □ **Really Well** □ **Just Okay**
□ **I'll Focus On Doing Better Tomorrow**

"Small steps equal big changes."

Daily Planner

Date: Weight:

Meals	What & How Much?	How was it prepared?	Where did you get your food?	Where did you eat?	Who did you eat with?
Breakfast					
Snack					
Lunch					

Snack

Dinner

**Dessert/
Snack**

Keepin' Hydrated!
8 x 8 ounces of water each day.

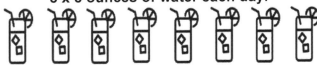

Exercise Today (Time & Type of Workouts)

What's Your Mood: Happy, quiet, sad, hopeful, bored, exhausted, lonely, peaceful, tired, stressed, joyful, calm?   **Make a note:**

What's My Day Been Like? Any Triggers? (Times, People, Moods, Situations)

What I Will Pay More Attention To: (Behaviors/Actions)

How Did I Do Today?

☐ **Brilliant**   ☐ **Really Well** ☐ **Just Okay**
☐ **I'll Focus On Doing Better Tomorrow**

"Be kind to yourself as well as others."

Daily Planner

Date: Weight:

Meals	What & How Much?	How was it prepared?	Where did you get your food?	Where did you eat?	Who did you eat with?
Breakfast					
Snack					
Lunch					

Snack

Dinner

**Dessert/
Snack**

Keepin' Hydrated!
8 x 8 ounces of water each day.

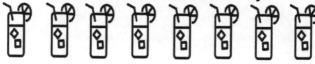

Exercise Today (Time & Type of Workouts)

What's Your Mood: Happy, quiet, sad, hopeful, bored, exhausted, lonely, peaceful, tired, stressed, joyful, calm?   **Make a note:**

What's My Day Been Like? Any Triggers? (Times, People, Moods, Situations)

What I Will Pay More Attention To: (Behaviors/Actions)

How Did I Do Today?

☐ **Brilliant**   ☐ **Really Well** ☐ **Just Okay**
☐ **I'll Focus On Doing Better Tomorrow**

"Every day is a new beginning."

Daily Planner

Date: Weight:

Meals	What & How Much?	How was it prepared?	Where did you get your food?	Where did you eat?	Who did you eat with?
Breakfast					
Snack					
Lunch					

Snack

Dinner

**Dessert/
Snack**

Keepin' Hydrated!
8 x 8 ounces of water each day.

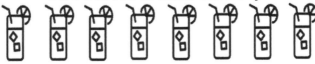

Exercise Today (Time & Type of Workouts)

What's Your Mood: Happy, quiet, sad, hopeful, bored, exhausted, lonely, peaceful, tired, stressed, joyful, calm?   **Make a note:**

What's My Day Been Like? Any Triggers? (Times, People, Moods, Situations)

What I Will Pay More Attention To: (Behaviors/Actions)

How Did I Do Today?

☐ **Brilliant**   ☐ **Really Well** ☐ **Just Okay**
☐ **I'll Focus On Doing Better Tomorrow**

"You are going great!"

Daily Planner

Date: Weight:

Meals	What & How Much?	How was it prepared?	Where did you get your food?	Where did you eat?	Who did you eat with?
Breakfast					
Snack					
Lunch					

Snack

Dinner

**Dessert/
Snack**

Keepin' Hydrated!
8 x 8 ounces of water each day.

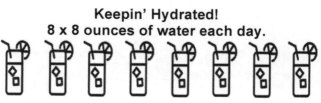

Exercise Today (Time & Type of Workouts)

What's Your Mood: Happy, quiet, sad, hopeful, bored, exhausted, lonely, peaceful, tired, stressed, joyful, calm?   **Make a note:**

What's My Day Been Like? Any Triggers? (Times, People, Moods, Situations)

What I Will Pay More Attention To: (Behaviors/Actions)

How Did I Do Today?

☐ **Brilliant**   ☐ **Really Well** ☐ **Just Okay**
☐ **I'll Focus On Doing Better Tomorrow**

"Every accomplishment starts with the willingness to try."

Daily Planner

Date: Weight:

Meals	What & How Much?	How was it prepared?	Where did you get your food?	Where did you eat?	Who did you eat with?
Breakfast					
Snack					
Lunch					

Snack

Dinner

**Dessert/
Snack**

Keepin' Hydrated!
8 x 8 ounces of water each day.

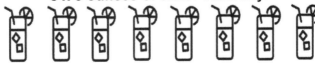

Exercise Today (Time & Type of Workouts)

What's Your Mood: Happy, quiet, sad, hopeful, bored, exhausted, lonely, peaceful, tired, stressed, joyful, calm?   **Make a note:**

What's My Day Been Like? Any Triggers? (Times, People, Moods, Situations)

What I Will Pay More Attention To: (Behaviors/Actions)

How Did I Do Today?

□ **Brilliant**   □ **Really Well** □ **Just Okay**
□ **I'll Focus On Doing Better Tomorrow**

"Just taking action is an accomplishment. Savor it"

Daily Planner

Date: Weight:

Meals	What & How Much?	How was it prepared?	Where did you get your food?	Where did you eat?	Who did you eat with?
Breakfast					
Snack					
Lunch					

Snack

Dinner

**Dessert/
Snack**

Keepin' Hydrated!
8 x 8 ounces of water each day.

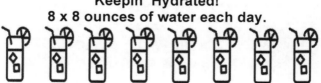

Exercise Today (Time & Type of Workouts)

What's Your Mood: Happy, quiet, sad, hopeful, bored, exhausted, lonely, peaceful, tired, stressed, joyful, calm?   **Make a note:**

What's My Day Been Like? Any Triggers? (Times, People, Moods, Situations)

What I Will Pay More Attention To: (Behaviors/Actions)

How Did I Do Today?

☐ **Brilliant**   ☐ **Really Well** ☐ **Just Okay**
☐ **I'll Focus On Doing Better Tomorrow**

"Take it a day at a time."

Daily Planner

Date: Weight:

Meals	What & How Much?	How was it prepared?	Where did you get your food?	Where did you eat?	Who did you eat with?
Breakfast					
Snack					
Lunch					

Snack

Dinner

**Dessert/
Snack**

Keepin' Hydrated!
8 x 8 ounces of water each day.

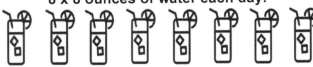

Exercise Today (Time & Type of Workouts)

What's Your Mood: Happy, quiet, sad, hopeful, bored, exhausted, lonely, peaceful, tired, stressed, joyful, calm?   **Make a note:**

What's My Day Been Like? Any Triggers? (Times, People, Moods, Situations)

What I Will Pay More Attention To: (Behaviors/Actions)

How Did I Do Today?

☐ **Brilliant**   ☐ **Really Well** ☐ **Just Okay**
☐ **I'll Focus On Doing Better Tomorrow**

"Every accomplishment starts with the willingness to try."

Daily Planner

Date: Weight:

Meals	What & How Much?	How was it prepared?	Where did you get your food?	Where did you eat?	Who did you eat with?
Breakfast					
Snack					
Lunch					

Snack

Dinner

**Dessert/
Snack**

Keepin' Hydrated!
8 x 8 ounces of water each day.

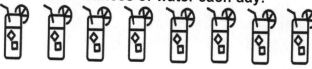

Exercise Today (Time & Type of Workouts)

What's Your Mood: Happy, quiet, sad, hopeful, bored, exhausted, lonely, peaceful, tired, stressed, joyful, calm?   **Make a note:**

What's My Day Been Like? Any Triggers? (Times, People, Moods, Situations)

What I Will Pay More Attention To: (Behaviors/Actions)

How Did I Do Today?

☐ **Brilliant**   ☐ **Really Well** ☐ **Just Okay**
☐ **I'll Focus On Doing Better Tomorrow**

"Every hour is precious. Be mindful of how you spend them."

Daily Planner

Date: Weight:

Meals	What & How Much?	How was it prepared?	Where did you get your food?	Where did you eat?	Who did you eat with?
Breakfast					
Snack					
Lunch					

Snack

Dinner

**Dessert/
Snack**

Keepin' Hydrated!
8 x 8 ounces of water each day.

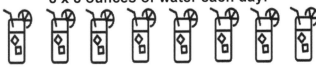

Exercise Today (Time & Type of Workouts)

What's Your Mood: Happy, quiet, sad, hopeful, bored, exhausted, lonely, peaceful, tired, stressed, joyful, calm?   **Make a note:**

What's My Day Been Like? Any Triggers? (Times, People, Moods, Situations)

What I Will Pay More Attention To: (Behaviors/Actions)

How Did I Do Today?

☐ **Brilliant**   ☐ **Really Well** ☐ **Just Okay**
☐ **I'll Focus On Doing Better Tomorrow**

"Every accomplishment starts with the willingness to try."

Daily Planner

Date: Weight:

Meals	What & How Much?	How was it prepared?	Where did you get your food?	Where did you eat?	Who did you eat with?
Breakfast					
Snack					
Lunch					

Snack

Dinner

**Dessert/
Snack**

Keepin' Hydrated!
8 x 8 ounces of water each day.

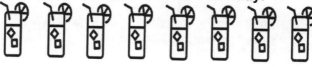

Exercise Today (Time & Type of Workouts)

What's Your Mood: Happy, quiet, sad, hopeful, bored, exhausted, lonely, peaceful, tired, stressed, joyful, calm?   **Make a note:**

What's My Day Been Like? Any Triggers? (Times, People, Moods, Situations)

What I Will Pay More Attention To: (Behaviors/Actions)

How Did I Do Today?

□ **Brilliant**   □ **Really Well** □ **Just Okay**
□ **I'll Focus On Doing Better Tomorrow**

"Try something new tomorrow."

Daily Planner

Date: Weight:

Meals	What & How Much?	How was it prepared?	Where did you get your food?	Where did you eat?	Who did you eat with?
Breakfast					
Snack					
Lunch					

Snack

Dinner

**Dessert/
Snack**

Keepin' Hydrated!
8 x 8 ounces of water each day.

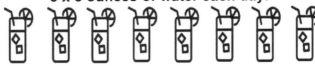

Exercise Today (Time & Type of Workouts)

What's Your Mood: Happy, quiet, sad, hopeful, bored, exhausted, lonely, peaceful, tired, stressed, joyful, calm?   **Make a note:**

What's My Day Been Like? Any Triggers? (Times, People, Moods, Situations)

What I Will Pay More Attention To: (Behaviors/Actions)

How Did I Do Today?

☐ **Brilliant**   ☐ **Really Well** ☐ **Just Okay**
☐ **I'll Focus On Doing Better Tomorrow**

"Look in the mirror and you will see a miracle."

Daily Planner

Date: _____ Weight: _____

Meals	What & How Much?	How was it prepared?	Where did you get your food?	Where did you eat?	Who did you eat with?
Breakfast					
Snack					
Lunch					

Snack

Dinner

**Dessert/
Snack**

Keepin' Hydrated!
8 x 8 ounces of water each day.

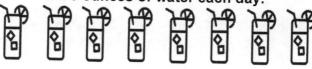

Exercise Today (Time & Type of Workouts)

What's Your Mood: Happy, quiet, sad, hopeful, bored, exhausted, lonely, peaceful, tired, stressed, joyful, calm?　　　**Make a note:**

What's My Day Been Like? Any Triggers? (Times, People, Moods, Situations)

What I Will Pay More Attention To: (Behaviors/Actions)

How Did I Do Today?

☐ **Brilliant**　　☐ **Really Well** ☐ **Just Okay**
☐ **I'll Focus On Doing Better Tomorrow**

"Listen to your favorite music and feel the joy."

Daily Planner

Date: Weight:

Meals	What & How Much?	How was it prepared?	Where did you get your food?	Where did you eat?	Who did you eat with?
Breakfast					
Snack					
Lunch					

Snack

Dinner

**Dessert/
Snack**

Keepin' Hydrated!
8 x 8 ounces of water each day.

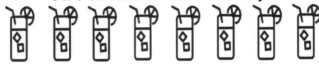

Exercise Today (Time & Type of Workouts)

What's Your Mood: Happy, quiet, sad, hopeful, bored, exhausted, lonely, peaceful, tired, stressed, joyful, calm?   Make a note:

What's My Day Been Like? Any Triggers? (Times, People, Moods, Situations)

What I Will Pay More Attention To: (Behaviors/Actions)

How Did I Do Today?

☐ **Brilliant**   ☐ **Really Well** ☐ **Just Okay**
☐ **I'll Focus On Doing Better Tomorrow**

"Every accomplishment starts with the willingness to try."

Daily Planner

Date: Weight:

Meals	What & How Much?	How was it prepared?	Where did you get your food?	Where did you eat?	Who did you eat with?
Breakfast					
Snack					
Lunch					

Snack

Dinner

**Dessert/
Snack**

Keepin' Hydrated!
8 x 8 ounces of water each day.

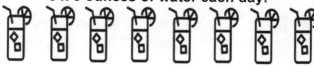

Exercise Today (Time & Type of Workouts)

What's Your Mood: Happy, quiet, sad, hopeful, bored, exhausted, lonely, peaceful, tired, stressed, joyful, calm?   **Make a note:**

What's My Day Been Like? Any Triggers? (Times, People, Moods, Situations)

What I Will Pay More Attention To: (Behaviors/Actions)

How Did I Do Today?

□ **Brilliant**   □ **Really Well** □ **Just Okay**
□ **I'll Focus On Doing Better Tomorrow**

"Every day is a new start."

Daily Planner

Date: Weight:

Meals	What & How Much?	How was it prepared?	Where did you get your food?	Where did you eat?	Who did you eat with?
Breakfast					
Snack					
Lunch					

Snack

Dinner

**Dessert/
Snack**

Keepin' Hydrated!
8 x 8 ounces of water each day.

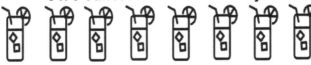

Exercise Today (Time & Type of Workouts)

What's Your Mood: Happy, quiet, sad, hopeful, bored, exhausted, lonely, peaceful, tired, stressed, joyful, calm?   **Make a note:**

What's My Day Been Like? Any Triggers? (Times, People, Moods, Situations)

What I Will Pay More Attention To: (Behaviors/Actions)

How Did I Do Today?

☐ **Brilliant**   ☐ **Really Well** ☐ **Just Okay**
☐ **I'll Focus On Doing Better Tomorrow**

"Every accomplishment starts with the willingness to try."

Daily Planner

Date: Weight:

Meals	What & How Much?	How was it prepared?	Where did you get your food?	Where did you eat?	Who did you eat with?
Breakfast					
Snack					
Lunch					

Snack

Dinner

**Dessert/
Snack**

Keepin' Hydrated!
8 x 8 ounces of water each day.

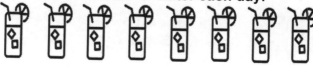

Exercise Today (Time & Type of Workouts)

What's Your Mood: Happy, quiet, sad, hopeful, bored, exhausted, lonely, peaceful, tired, stressed, joyful, calm?   **Make a note:**

What's My Day Been Like? Any Triggers? (Times, People, Moods, Situations)

What I Will Pay More Attention To: (Behaviors/Actions)

How Did I Do Today?

☐ **Brilliant**   ☐ **Really Well** ☐ **Just Okay**
☐ **I'll Focus On Doing Better Tomorrow**

"Good habits are built on small steps."

Daily Planner

Date: Weight:

Meals	What & How Much?	How was it prepared?	Where did you get your food?	Where did you eat?	Who did you eat with?
Breakfast					
Snack					
Lunch					

Snack

Dinner

**Dessert/
Snack**

Keepin' Hydrated!
8 x 8 ounces of water each day.

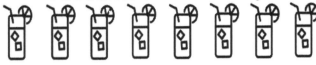

Exercise Today (Time & Type of Workouts)

What's Your Mood: Happy, quiet, sad, hopeful, bored, exhausted, lonely, peaceful, tired, stressed, joyful, calm?　　　　**Make a note:**

What's My Day Been Like? Any Triggers? (Times, People, Moods, Situations)

What I Will Pay More Attention To: (Behaviors/Actions)

How Did I Do Today?

□ **Brilliant**　　□ **Really Well** □ **Just Okay**
□ **I'll Focus On Doing Better Tomorrow**

"Keep going!"

Daily Planner

Date: Weight:

Meals	What & How Much?	How was it prepared?	Where did you get your food?	Where did you eat?	Who did you eat with?
Breakfast					
Snack					
Lunch					

Snack

Dinner

**Dessert/
Snack**

Keepin' Hydrated!
8 x 8 ounces of water each day.

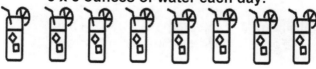

Exercise Today (Time & Type of Workouts)

What's Your Mood: Happy, quiet, sad, hopeful, bored, exhausted, lonely, peaceful, tired, stressed, joyful, calm? **Make a note:**

What's My Day Been Like? Any Triggers? (Times, People, Moods, Situations)

What I Will Pay More Attention To: (Behaviors/Actions)

How Did I Do Today?

□ **Brilliant**   □ **Really Well** □ **Just Okay**
□ **I'll Focus On Doing Better Tomorrow**

"Every accomplishment starts with the willingness to try."

Daily Planner

Date: Weight:

Meals	What & How Much?	How was it prepared?	Where did you get your food?	Where did you eat?	Who did you eat with?
Breakfast					
Snack					
Lunch					

Snack

Dinner

**Dessert/
Snack**

Keepin' Hydrated!
8 x 8 ounces of water each day.

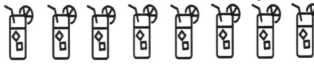

Exercise Today (Time & Type of Workouts)

What's Your Mood: Happy, quiet, sad, hopeful, bored, exhausted, lonely, peaceful, tired, stressed, joyful, calm?　　　**Make a note:**

What's My Day Been Like? Any Triggers? (Times, People, Moods, Situations)

What I Will Pay More Attention To: (Behaviors/Actions)

How Did I Do Today?

☐ **Brilliant**　　☐ **Really Well** ☐ **Just Okay**
☐ **I'll Focus On Doing Better Tomorrow**

"Expect success and a healthy tomorrow."

Daily Planner

Date: Weight:

Meals	What & How Much?	How was it prepared?	Where did you get your food?	Where did you eat?	Who did you eat with?
Breakfast					
Snack					
Lunch					

Snack

Dinner

**Dessert/
Snack**

Keepin' Hydrated!
8 x 8 ounces of water each day.

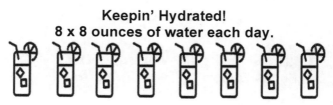

Exercise Today (Time & Type of Workouts)

What's Your Mood: Happy, quiet, sad, hopeful, bored, exhausted, lonely, peaceful, tired, stressed, joyful, calm?   **Make a note:**

What's My Day Been Like? Any Triggers? (Times, People, Moods, Situations)

What I Will Pay More Attention To: (Behaviors/Actions)

How Did I Do Today?

☐ **Brilliant**   ☐ **Really Well** ☐ **Just Okay**
☐ **I'll Focus On Doing Better Tomorrow**

"Have a willingness to take action."

Daily Planner

Date: Weight:

Meals	What & How Much?	How was it prepared?	Where did you get your food?	Where did you eat?	Who did you eat with?
Breakfast					
Snack					
Lunch					

Snack

Dinner

**Dessert/
Snack**

Keepin' Hydrated!
8 x 8 ounces of water each day.

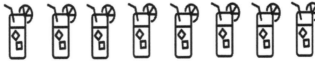

Exercise Today (Time & Type of Workouts)

What's Your Mood: Happy, quiet, sad, hopeful, bored, exhausted, lonely, peaceful, tired, stressed, joyful, calm?   **Make a note:**

What's My Day Been Like? Any Triggers? (Times, People, Moods, Situations)

What I Will Pay More Attention To: (Behaviors/Actions)

How Did I Do Today?

☐ **Brilliant**   ☐ **Really Well** ☐ **Just Okay**
☐ **I'll Focus On Doing Better Tomorrow**

"Every accomplishment starts with the willingness to try."

Daily Planner

Date: Weight:

Meals	What & How Much?	How was it prepared?	Where did you get your food?	Where did you eat?	Who did you eat with?
Breakfast					
Snack					
Lunch					

Snack

Dinner

**Dessert/
Snack**

Keepin' Hydrated!
8 x 8 ounces of water each day.

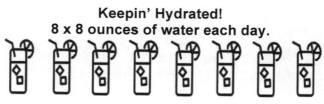

Exercise Today (Time & Type of Workouts)

What's Your Mood: Happy, quiet, sad, hopeful, bored, exhausted, lonely, peaceful, tired, stressed, joyful, calm?   **Make a note:**

What's My Day Been Like? Any Triggers? (Times, People, Moods, Situations)

What I Will Pay More Attention To: (Behaviors/Actions)

How Did I Do Today?

□ **Brilliant**   □ **Really Well** □ **Just Okay**
□ **I'll Focus On Doing Better Tomorrow**

"Be as kind to yourself as you are to others."

Daily Planner

Date: Weight:

Meals	What & How Much?	How was it prepared?	Where did you get your food?	Where did you eat?	Who did you eat with?
Breakfast					
Snack					
Lunch					

Snack

Dinner

**Dessert/
Snack**

Keepin' Hydrated!
8 x 8 ounces of water each day.

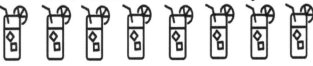

Exercise Today (Time & Type of Workouts)

What's Your Mood: Happy, quiet, sad, hopeful, bored, exhausted, lonely, peaceful, tired, stressed, joyful, calm? **Make a note:**

What's My Day Been Like? Any Triggers? (Times, People, Moods, Situations)

What I Will Pay More Attention To: (Behaviors/Actions)

How Did I Do Today?

☐ **Brilliant**   ☐ **Really Well** ☐ **Just Okay**
☐ **I'll Focus On Doing Better Tomorrow**

"Every accomplishment starts with the willingness to try."

Daily Planner

Date: Weight:

Meals	What & How Much?	How was it prepared?	Where did you get your food?	Where did you eat?	Who did you eat with?
Breakfast					
Snack					
Lunch					

Snack

Dinner

**Dessert/
Snack**

Keepin' Hydrated!
8 x 8 ounces of water each day.

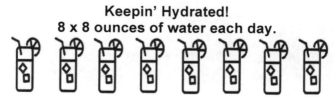

Exercise Today (Time & Type of Workouts)

What's Your Mood: Happy, quiet, sad, hopeful, bored, exhausted, lonely, peaceful, tired, stressed, joyful, calm?   **Make a note:**

What's My Day Been Like? Any Triggers? (Times, People, Moods, Situations)

What I Will Pay More Attention To: (Behaviors/Actions)

How Did I Do Today?

□ **Brilliant**   □ **Really Well** □ **Just Okay**
□ **I'll Focus On Doing Better Tomorrow**

"And tomorrow is another opportunity to start again."

Daily Planner

Date: Weight:

Meals	What & How Much?	How was it prepared?	Where did you get your food?	Where did you eat?	Who did you eat with?
Breakfast					
Snack					
Lunch					

Snack

Dinner

**Dessert/
Snack**

Keepin' Hydrated!
8 x 8 ounces of water each day.

Exercise Today (Time & Type of Workouts)

What's Your Mood: Happy, quiet, sad, hopeful, bored, exhausted, lonely, peaceful, tired, stressed, joyful, calm?   **Make a note:**

What's My Day Been Like? Any Triggers? (Times, People, Moods, Situations)

What I Will Pay More Attention To: (Behaviors/Actions)

How Did I Do Today?

☐ **Brilliant**   ☐ **Really Well** ☐ **Just Okay**
☐ **I'll Focus On Doing Better Tomorrow**

"Every accomplishment starts with the willingness to try."

Daily Planner

Date: Weight:

Meals	What & How Much?	How was it prepared?	Where did you get your food?	Where did you eat?	Who did you eat with?
Breakfast					
Snack					
Lunch					

Snack

Dinner

**Dessert/
Snack**

Keepin' Hydrated!
8 x 8 ounces of water each day.

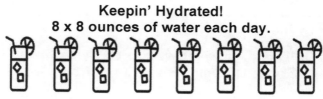

Exercise Today (Time & Type of Workouts)

What's Your Mood: Happy, quiet, sad, hopeful, bored, exhausted, lonely, peaceful, tired, stressed, joyful, calm? **Make a note:**

What's My Day Been Like? Any Triggers? (Times, People, Moods, Situations)

What I Will Pay More Attention To: (Behaviors/Actions)

How Did I Do Today?

☐ **Brilliant**   ☐ **Really Well** ☐ **Just Okay**
☐ **I'll Focus On Doing Better Tomorrow**

"Every step equals action. Action is growth."

Daily Planner

Date: _____   Weight: _____

Meals	What & How Much?	How was it prepared?	Where did you get your food?	Where did you eat?	Who did you eat with?
Breakfast					
Snack					
Lunch					

Snack

Dinner

**Dessert/
Snack**

Keepin' Hydrated!
8 x 8 ounces of water each day.

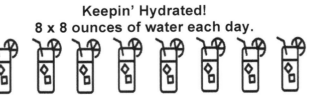

Exercise Today (Time & Type of Workouts)

What's Your Mood: Happy, quiet, sad, hopeful, bored, exhausted, lonely, peaceful, tired, stressed, joyful, calm?   **Make a note:**

What's My Day Been Like? Any Triggers? (Times, People, Moods, Situations)

What I Will Pay More Attention To: (Behaviors/Actions)

How Did I Do Today?

☐ **Brilliant**   ☐ **Really Well** ☐ **Just Okay**
☐ **I'll Focus On Doing Better Tomorrow**

"We all make mistakes. Will you let them stop or motivate you?"

Daily Planner

Date: _____   Weight: _____

Meals	What & How Much?	How was it prepared?	Where did you get your food?	Where did you eat?	Who did you eat with?
Breakfast					
Snack					
Lunch					

Snack

Dinner

**Dessert/
Snack**

Keepin' Hydrated!
8 x 8 ounces of water each day.

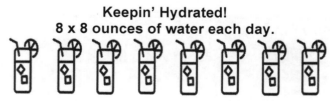

Exercise Today (Time & Type of Workouts)

What's Your Mood: Happy, quiet, sad, hopeful, bored, exhausted, lonely, peaceful, tired, stressed, joyful, calm?   Make a note:

What's My Day Been Like? Any Triggers? (Times, People, Moods, Situations)

What I Will Pay More Attention To: (Behaviors/Actions)

How Did I Do Today?

□ **Brilliant**   □ **Really Well** □ **Just Okay**
□ **I'll Focus On Doing Better Tomorrow**

"Every accomplishment starts with the willingness to try."

Daily Planner

Date: Weight:

Meals	What & How Much?	How was it prepared?	Where did you get your food?	Where did you eat?	Who did you eat with?
Breakfast					
Snack					
Lunch					

Snack

Dinner

**Dessert/
Snack**

Keepin' Hydrated!
8 x 8 ounces of water each day.

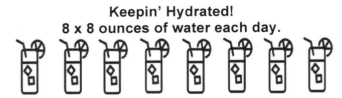

Exercise Today (Time & Type of Workouts)

What's Your Mood: Happy, quiet, sad, hopeful, bored, exhausted, lonely, peaceful, tired, stressed, joyful, calm?   **Make a note:**

What's My Day Been Like? Any Triggers? (Times, People, Moods, Situations)

What I Will Pay More Attention To: (Behaviors/Actions)

How Did I Do Today?

☐ **Brilliant**   ☐ **Really Well** ☐ **Just Okay**
☐ **I'll Focus On Doing Better Tomorrow**

"Every day is a new beginning."

Daily Planner

Date: _____   Weight: _____

Meals	What & How Much?	How was it prepared?	Where did you get your food?	Where did you eat?	Who did you eat with?
Breakfast					
Snack					
Lunch					

Snack

Dinner

**Dessert/
Snack**

Keepin' Hydrated!
8 x 8 ounces of water each day.

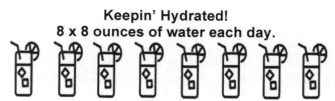

Exercise Today (Time & Type of Workouts)

What's Your Mood: Happy, quiet, sad, hopeful, bored, exhausted, lonely, peaceful, tired, stressed, joyful, calm?   **Make a note:**

What's My Day Been Like? Any Triggers? (Times, People, Moods, Situations)

What I Will Pay More Attention To: (Behaviors/Actions)

How Did I Do Today?

☐ **Brilliant**   ☐ **Really Well** ☐ **Just Okay**
☐ **I'll Focus On Doing Better Tomorrow**

"Keep going!"

Daily Planner

Date: Weight:

Meals	What & How Much?	How was it prepared?	Where did you get your food?	Where did you eat?	Who did you eat with?
Breakfast					
Snack					
Lunch					

Snack

Dinner

**Dessert/
Snack**

Keepin' Hydrated!
8 x 8 ounces of water each day.

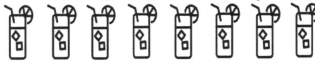

Exercise Today (Time & Type of Workouts)

What's Your Mood: Happy, quiet, sad, hopeful, bored, exhausted, lonely, peaceful, tired, stressed, joyful, calm?   **Make a note:**

What's My Day Been Like? Any Triggers? (Times, People, Moods, Situations)

What I Will Pay More Attention To: (Behaviors/Actions)

How Did I Do Today?

□ **Brilliant**   □ **Really Well** □ **Just Okay**
□ **I'll Focus On Doing Better Tomorrow**

"Remember, you've got this."

Daily Planner

Date: Weight:

Meals	What & How Much?	How was it prepared?	Where did you get your food?	Where did you eat?	Who did you eat with?
Breakfast					
Snack					
Lunch					

Snack

Dinner

**Dessert/
Snack**

Keepin' Hydrated!
8 x 8 ounces of water each day.

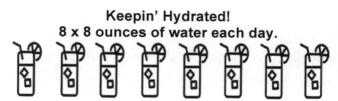

Exercise Today (Time & Type of Workouts)

What's Your Mood: Happy, quiet, sad, hopeful, bored, exhausted, lonely, peaceful, tired, stressed, joyful, calm?   **Make a note:**

What's My Day Been Like? Any Triggers? (Times, People, Moods, Situations)

What I Will Pay More Attention To: (Behaviors/Actions)

How Did I Do Today?

☐ **Brilliant**   ☐ **Really Well** ☐ **Just Okay**
☐ **I'll Focus On Doing Better Tomorrow**

"Be gentle with yourself and expect success."

Daily Planner

Date: Weight:

Meals	What & How Much?	How was it prepared?	Where did you get your food?	Where did you eat?	Who did you eat with?
Breakfast					
Snack					
Lunch					

Snack

Dinner

**Dessert/
Snack**

Keepin' Hydrated!
8 x 8 ounces of water each day.

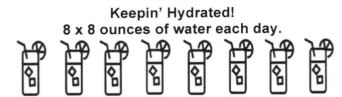

Exercise Today (Time & Type of Workouts)

What's Your Mood: Happy, quiet, sad, hopeful, bored, exhausted, lonely, peaceful, tired, stressed, joyful, calm?   **Make a note:**

What's My Day Been Like? Any Triggers? (Times, People, Moods, Situations)

What I Will Pay More Attention To: (Behaviors/Actions)

How Did I Do Today?

☐ **Brilliant**   ☐ **Really Well** ☐ **Just Okay**
☐ **I'll Focus On Doing Better Tomorrow**

"New healthy habits start with small steps."

Daily Planner

Date: _____ Weight: _____

Meals	What & How Much?	How was it prepared?	Where did you get your food?	Where did you eat?	Who did you eat with?
Breakfast					
Snack					
Lunch					

Snack

Dinner

**Dessert/
Snack**

Keepin' Hydrated!
8 x 8 ounces of water each day.

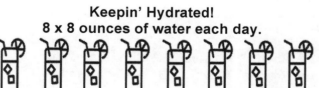

Exercise Today (Time & Type of Workouts)

What's Your Mood: Happy, quiet, sad, hopeful, bored, exhausted, lonely, peaceful, tired, stressed, joyful, calm?   **Make a note:**

What's My Day Been Like? Any Triggers? (Times, People, Moods, Situations)

What I Will Pay More Attention To: (Behaviors/Actions)

How Did I Do Today?

☐ **Brilliant**   ☐ **Really Well** ☐ **Just Okay**
☐ **I'll Focus On Doing Better Tomorrow**

"Every accomplishment starts with the willingness to try."

Daily Planner

Date: Weight:

Meals	What & How Much?	How was it prepared?	Where did you get your food?	Where did you eat?	Who did you eat with?
Breakfast					
Snack					
Lunch					

Snack

Dinner

**Dessert/
Snack**

Keepin' Hydrated!
8 x 8 ounces of water each day.

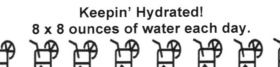
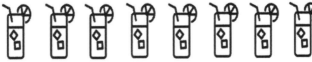

Exercise Today (Time & Type of Workouts)

What's Your Mood: Happy, quiet, sad, hopeful, bored, exhausted, lonely, peaceful, tired, stressed, joyful, calm?   **Make a note:**

What's My Day Been Like? Any Triggers? (Times, People, Moods, Situations)

What I Will Pay More Attention To: (Behaviors/Actions)

How Did I Do Today?

☐ **Brilliant**   ☐ **Really Well** ☐ **Just Okay**
☐ **I'll Focus On Doing Better Tomorrow**

"Pay attention to how your food tastes."

Daily Planner

Date: _____ Weight: _____

Meals	What & How Much?	How was it prepared?	Where did you get your food?	Where did you eat?	Who did you eat with?
Breakfast					
Snack					
Lunch					

Snack

Dinner

Dessert/
Snack

Keepin' Hydrated!
8 x 8 ounces of water each day.

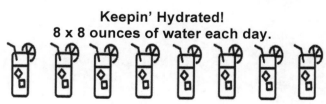

Exercise Today (Time & Type of Workouts)

What's Your Mood: Happy, quiet, sad, hopeful, bored, exhausted, lonely, peaceful, tired, stressed, joyful, calm?   **Make a note:**

What's My Day Been Like? Any Triggers? (Times, People, Moods, Situations)

What I Will Pay More Attention To: (Behaviors/Actions)

How Did I Do Today?

☐ **Brilliant**   ☐ **Really Well** ☐ **Just Okay**
☐ **I'll Focus On Doing Better Tomorrow**

"Keep at it!"

Daily Planner

Date: _____ Weight: _____

Meals	What & How Much?	How was it prepared?	Where did you get your food?	Where did you eat?	Who did you eat with?
Breakfast					
Snack					
Lunch					

Snack

Dinner

**Dessert/
Snack**

Keepin' Hydrated!
8 x 8 ounces of water each day.

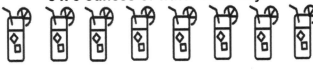

Exercise Today (Time & Type of Workouts)

What's Your Mood: Happy, quiet, sad, hopeful, bored, exhausted, lonely, peaceful, tired, stressed, joyful, calm?   **Make a note:**

What's My Day Been Like? Any Triggers? (Times, People, Moods, Situations)

What I Will Pay More Attention To: (Behaviors/Actions)

How Did I Do Today?

□ **Brilliant**   □ **Really Well** □ **Just Okay**
□ **I'll Focus On Doing Better Tomorrow**

"Every accomplishment starts with small steps."

Daily Planner

Date: Weight:

Meals	What & How Much?	How was it prepared?	Where did you get your food?	Where did you eat?	Who did you eat with?
Breakfast					
Snack					
Lunch					

Snack

Dinner

**Dessert/
Snack**

Keepin' Hydrated!
8 x 8 ounces of water each day.

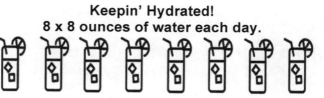

Exercise Today (Time & Type of Workouts)

What's Your Mood: Happy, quiet, sad, hopeful, bored, exhausted, lonely, peaceful, tired, stressed, joyful, calm?   Make a note:

What's My Day Been Like? Any Triggers? (Times, People, Moods, Situations)

What I Will Pay More Attention To: (Behaviors/Actions)

How Did I Do Today?

☐ **Brilliant**   ☐ **Really Well** ☐ **Just Okay**
☐ **I'll Focus On Doing Better Tomorrow**

"Every accomplishment starts with the willingness to try."

Daily Planner

Date: Weight:

Meals	What & How Much?	How was it prepared?	Where did you get your food?	Where did you eat?	Who did you eat with?
Breakfast					
Snack					
Lunch					

Snack

Dinner

**Dessert/
Snack**

Keepin' Hydrated!
8 x 8 ounces of water each day.

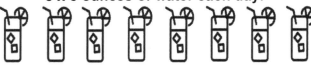

Exercise Today (Time & Type of Workouts)

What's Your Mood: Happy, quiet, sad, hopeful, bored, exhausted, lonely, peaceful, tired, stressed, joyful, calm?   **Make a note:**

What's My Day Been Like? Any Triggers? (Times, People, Moods, Situations)

What I Will Pay More Attention To: (Behaviors/Actions)

How Did I Do Today?

☐ **Brilliant**   ☐ **Really Well** ☐ **Just Okay**
☐ **I'll Focus On Doing Better Tomorrow**

"Just take it a day at a time."

Daily Planner

Date: Weight:

Meals	What & How Much?	How was it prepared?	Where did you get your food?	Where did you eat?	Who did you eat with?
Breakfast					
Snack					
Lunch					

Snack

Dinner

**Dessert/
Snack**

Keepin' Hydrated!
8 x 8 ounces of water each day.

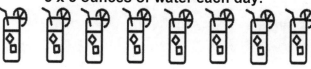

Exercise Today (Time & Type of Workouts)

What's Your Mood: Happy, quiet, sad, hopeful, bored, exhausted, lonely, peaceful, tired, stressed, joyful, calm?   **Make a note:**

What's My Day Been Like? Any Triggers? (Times, People, Moods, Situations)

What I Will Pay More Attention To: (Behaviors/Actions)

How Did I Do Today?

☐ **Brilliant**   ☐ **Really Well** ☐ **Just Okay**
☐ **I'll Focus On Doing Better Tomorrow**

"Small steps equal big changes."

Daily Planner

Date: Weight:

Meals	What & How Much?	How was it prepared?	Where did you get your food?	Where did you eat?	Who did you eat with?
Breakfast					
Snack					
Lunch					

Snack

Dinner

**Dessert/
Snack**

Keepin' Hydrated!
8 x 8 ounces of water each day.

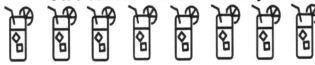

Exercise Today (Time & Type of Workouts)

What's Your Mood: Happy, quiet, sad, hopeful, bored, exhausted, lonely, peaceful, tired, stressed, joyful, calm?   **Make a note:**

What's My Day Been Like? Any Triggers? (Times, People, Moods, Situations)

What I Will Pay More Attention To: (Behaviors/Actions)

How Did I Do Today?

□ **Brilliant**   □ **Really Well** □ **Just Okay**
□ **I'll Focus On Doing Better Tomorrow**

"Every accomplishment starts with the willingness to try."

Daily Planner

Date: Weight:

Meals	What & How Much?	How was it prepared?	Where did you get your food?	Where did you eat?	Who did you eat with?
Breakfast					
Snack					
Lunch					

Snack

Dinner

**Dessert/
Snack**

Keepin' Hydrated!
8 x 8 ounces of water each day.

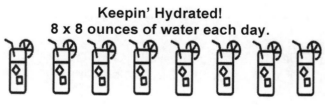

Exercise Today (Time & Type of Workouts)

What's Your Mood: Happy, quiet, sad, hopeful, bored, exhausted, lonely, peaceful, tired, stressed, joyful, calm?   **Make a note:**

What's My Day Been Like? Any Triggers? (Times, People, Moods, Situations)

What I Will Pay More Attention To: (Behaviors/Actions)

How Did I Do Today?

☐ **Brilliant**   ☐ **Really Well** ☐ **Just Okay**
☐ **I'll Focus On Doing Better Tomorrow**

"Every change can be met with your determination."

Daily Planner

Date: Weight:

Meals	What & How Much?	How was it prepared?	Where did you get your food?	Where did you eat?	Who did you eat with?
Breakfast					
Snack					
Lunch					

Snack

Dinner

**Dessert/
Snack**

Keepin' Hydrated!
8 x 8 ounces of water each day.

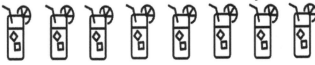

Exercise Today (Time & Type of Workouts)

What's Your Mood: Happy, quiet, sad, hopeful, bored, exhausted, lonely, peaceful, tired, stressed, joyful, calm?   **Make a note:**

What's My Day Been Like? Any Triggers? (Times, People, Moods, Situations)

What I Will Pay More Attention To: (Behaviors/Actions)

How Did I Do Today?

☐ **Brilliant**   ☐ **Really Well** ☐ **Just Okay**
☐ **I'll Focus On Doing Better Tomorrow**

"Change is uncomfortable at first, but soon it becomes habit."

Daily Planner

Date: Weight:

Meals	What & How Much?	How was it prepared?	Where did you get your food?	Where did you eat?	Who did you eat with?
Breakfast					
Snack					
Lunch					

Snack

Dinner

**Dessert/
Snack**

Keepin' Hydrated!
8 x 8 ounces of water each day.

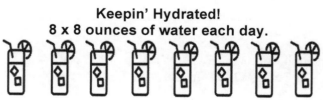

Exercise Today (Time & Type of Workouts)

What's Your Mood: Happy, quiet, sad, hopeful, bored, exhausted, lonely, peaceful, tired, stressed, joyful, calm?   **Make a note:**

What's My Day Been Like? Any Triggers? (Times, People, Moods, Situations)

What I Will Pay More Attention To: (Behaviors/Actions)

How Did I Do Today?

☐ **Brilliant**   ☐ **Really Well** ☐ **Just Okay**
☐ **I'll Focus On Doing Better Tomorrow**

"Every accomplishment starts with the willingness to try."

Daily Planner

Date: Weight:

Meals	What & How Much?	How was it prepared?	Where did you get your food?	Where did you eat?	Who did you eat with?
Breakfast					
Snack					
Lunch					

Snack

Dinner

**Dessert/
Snack**

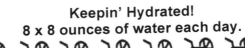

Keepin' Hydrated!
8 x 8 ounces of water each day.

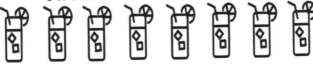

Exercise Today (Time & Type of Workouts)

What's Your Mood: Happy, quiet, sad, hopeful, bored, exhausted, lonely, peaceful, tired, stressed, joyful, calm?   **Make a note:**

What's My Day Been Like? Any Triggers? (Times, People, Moods, Situations)

What I Will Pay More Attention To: (Behaviors/Actions)

How Did I Do Today?

☐ **Brilliant**   ☐ **Really Well** ☐ **Just Okay**
☐ **I'll Focus On Doing Better Tomorrow**

"Take it a day at a time."

Daily Planner

Date: Weight:

Meals	What & How Much?	How was it prepared?	Where did you get your food?	Where did you eat?	Who did you eat with?
Breakfast					
Snack					
Lunch					

Snack

Dinner

**Dessert/
Snack**

Keepin' Hydrated!
8 x 8 ounces of water each day.

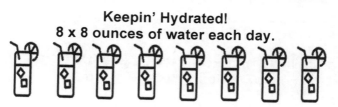

Exercise Today (Time & Type of Workouts)

What's Your Mood: Happy, quiet, sad, hopeful, bored, exhausted, lonely, peaceful, tired, stressed, joyful, calm?   **Make a note:**

What's My Day Been Like? Any Triggers? (Times, People, Moods, Situations)

What I Will Pay More Attention To: (Behaviors/Actions)

How Did I Do Today?

☐ **Brilliant**   ☐ **Really Well** ☐ **Just Okay**
☐ **I'll Focus On Doing Better Tomorrow**

"You've got this!"

Daily Planner

Date: Weight:

Meals	What & How Much?	How was it prepared?	Where did you get your food?	Where did you eat?	Who did you eat with?
Breakfast					
Snack					
Lunch					

Snack

Dinner

**Dessert/
Snack**

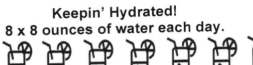

Keepin' Hydrated!
8 x 8 ounces of water each day.

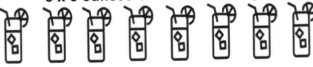

Exercise Today (Time & Type of Workouts)

What's Your Mood: Happy, quiet, sad, hopeful, bored, exhausted, lonely, peaceful, tired, stressed, joyful, calm? **Make a note:**

What's My Day Been Like? Any Triggers? (Times, People, Moods, Situations)

What I Will Pay More Attention To: (Behaviors/Actions)

How Did I Do Today?

☐ **Brilliant**   ☐ **Really Well** ☐ **Just Okay**
☐ **I'll Focus On Doing Better Tomorrow**

"Small steps equal big changes."

Daily Planner

Date: Weight:

Meals	What & How Much?	How was it prepared?	Where did you get your food?	Where did you eat?	Who did you eat with?
Breakfast					
Snack					
Lunch					

Snack

Dinner

**Dessert/
Snack**

Keepin' Hydrated!
8 x 8 ounces of water each day.

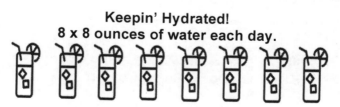

Exercise Today (Time & Type of Workouts)

What's Your Mood: Happy, quiet, sad, hopeful, bored, exhausted, lonely, peaceful, tired, stressed, joyful, calm?   **Make a note:**

What's My Day Been Like? Any Triggers? (Times, People, Moods, Situations)

What I Will Pay More Attention To: (Behaviors/Actions)

How Did I Do Today?

☐ **Brilliant**   ☐ **Really Well** ☐ **Just Okay**
☐ **I'll Focus On Doing Better Tomorrow**

"Accept that you will be successful."

Daily Planner

Date: Weight:

Meals	What & How Much?	How was it prepared?	Where did you get your food?	Where did you eat?	Who did you eat with?
Breakfast					
Snack					
Lunch					

Snack

Dinner

**Dessert/
Snack**

Keepin' Hydrated!
8 x 8 ounces of water each day.

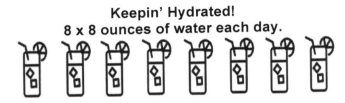

Exercise Today (Time & Type of Workouts)

What's Your Mood: Happy, quiet, sad, hopeful, bored, exhausted, lonely, peaceful, tired, stressed, joyful, calm?   **Make a note:**

**What's My Day Been Like? Any Triggers?
(Times, People, Moods, Situations)**

**What I Will Pay More Attention To:
(Behaviors/Actions)**

How Did I Do Today?

☐ **Brilliant**   ☐ **Really Well** ☐ **Just Okay**
☐ **I'll Focus On Doing Better Tomorrow**

"Every accomplishment starts with the willingness to try."

Daily Planner

Date: Weight:

Meals	What & How Much?	How was it prepared?	Where did you get your food?	Where did you eat?	Who did you eat with?
Breakfast					
Snack					
Lunch					

Snack

Dinner

**Dessert/
Snack**

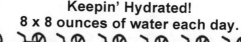

Keepin' Hydrated!
8 x 8 ounces of water each day.

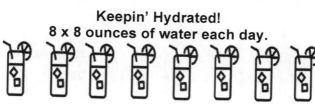

Exercise Today (Time & Type of Workouts)

What's Your Mood: Happy, quiet, sad, hopeful, bored, exhausted, lonely, peaceful, tired, stressed, joyful, calm? **Make a note:**

What's My Day Been Like? Any Triggers? (Times, People, Moods, Situations)

What I Will Pay More Attention To: (Behaviors/Actions)

How Did I Do Today?

☐ **Brilliant**   ☐ **Really Well** ☐ **Just Okay**
☐ **I'll Focus On Doing Better Tomorrow**

"Expect and accept all that is good around you."

Daily Planner

Date: Weight:

Meals	What & How Much?	How was it prepared?	Where did you get your food?	Where did you eat?	Who did you eat with?
Breakfast					
Snack					
Lunch					

Snack

Dinner

**Dessert/
Snack**

Keepin' Hydrated!
8 x 8 ounces of water each day.

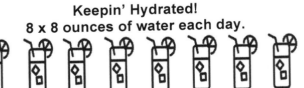

Exercise Today (Time & Type of Workouts)

What's Your Mood: Happy, quiet, sad, hopeful, bored, exhausted, lonely, peaceful, tired, stressed, joyful, calm?   **Make a note:**

What's My Day Been Like? Any Triggers? (Times, People, Moods, Situations)

What I Will Pay More Attention To: (Behaviors/Actions)

How Did I Do Today?

☐ **Brilliant**   ☐ **Really Well** ☐ **Just Okay**
☐ **I'll Focus On Doing Better Tomorrow**

"Every accomplishment starts with the willingness to try."

Daily Planner

Date: _____   Weight: _____

Meals	What & How Much?	How was it prepared?	Where did you get your food?	Where did you eat?	Who did you eat with?
Breakfast					
Snack					
Lunch					

Snack

Dinner

**Dessert/
Snack**

Keepin' Hydrated!
8 x 8 ounces of water each day.

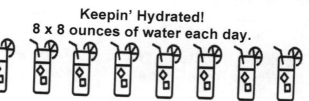

Exercise Today (Time & Type of Workouts)

What's Your Mood: Happy, quiet, sad, hopeful, bored, exhausted, lonely, peaceful, tired, stressed, joyful, calm? Make a note:

What's My Day Been Like? Any Triggers? (Times, People, Moods, Situations)

What I Will Pay More Attention To: (Behaviors/Actions)

How Did I Do Today?

☐ **Brilliant** ☐ **Really Well** ☐ **Just Okay**
☐ **I'll Focus On Doing Better Tomorrow**

"You've got this."

Daily Planner

Date: Weight:

Meals	What & How Much?	How was it prepared?	Where did you get your food?	Where did you eat?	Who did you eat with?
Breakfast					
Snack					
Lunch					

Snack

Dinner

**Dessert/
Snack**

Keepin' Hydrated!
8 x 8 ounces of water each day.

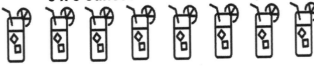

Exercise Today (Time & Type of Workouts)

What's Your Mood: Happy, quiet, sad, hopeful, bored, exhausted, lonely, peaceful, tired, stressed, joyful, calm?   **Make a note:**

What's My Day Been Like? Any Triggers? (Times, People, Moods, Situations)

What I Will Pay More Attention To: (Behaviors/Actions)

How Did I Do Today?

☐ **Brilliant**   ☐ **Really Well** ☐ **Just Okay**
☐ **I'll Focus On Doing Better Tomorrow**

"Every accomplishment starts with the willingness to try."

Daily Planner

Date: _____   Weight: _____

Meals	What & How Much?	How was it prepared?	Where did you get your food?	Where did you eat?	Who did you eat with?
Breakfast					
Snack					
Lunch					

Snack

Dinner

**Dessert/
Snack**

Keepin' Hydrated!
8 x 8 ounces of water each day.

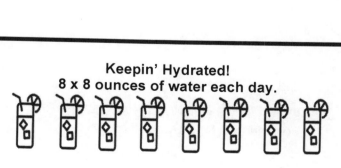

Exercise Today (Time & Type of Workouts)

What's Your Mood: Happy, quiet, sad, hopeful, bored, exhausted, lonely, peaceful, tired, stressed, joyful, calm?   **Make a note:**

What's My Day Been Like? Any Triggers? (Times, People, Moods, Situations)

What I Will Pay More Attention To: (Behaviors/Actions)

How Did I Do Today?

☐ **Brilliant**   ☐ **Really Well** ☐ **Just Okay**
☐ **I'll Focus On Doing Better Tomorrow**

"Every new day is a chance to begin again."

Daily Planner

Date: Weight:

Meals	What & How Much?	How was it prepared?	Where did you get your food?	Where did you eat?	Who did you eat with?
Breakfast					
Snack					
Lunch					

Snack

Dinner

**Dessert/
Snack**

Keepin' Hydrated!
8 x 8 ounces of water each day.

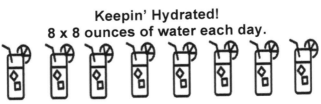

Exercise Today (Time & Type of Workouts)

What's Your Mood: Happy, quiet, sad, hopeful, bored, exhausted, lonely, peaceful, tired, stressed, joyful, calm?   **Make a note:**

What's My Day Been Like? Any Triggers? (Times, People, Moods, Situations)

What I Will Pay More Attention To: (Behaviors/Actions)

How Did I Do Today?

☐ **Brilliant**   ☐ **Really Well** ☐ **Just Okay**
☐ **I'll Focus On Doing Better Tomorrow**

"You are more special than you know."

Daily Planner

Date: Weight:

Meals	What & How Much?	How was it prepared?	Where did you get your food?	Where did you eat?	Who did you eat with?
Breakfast					
Snack					
Lunch					

Snack

Dinner

**Dessert/
Snack**

Keepin' Hydrated!
8 x 8 ounces of water each day.

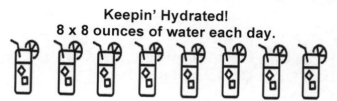

Exercise Today (Time & Type of Workouts)

What's Your Mood: Happy, quiet, sad, hopeful, bored, exhausted, lonely, peaceful, tired, stressed, joyful, calm?   **Make a note:**

What's My Day Been Like? Any Triggers? (Times, People, Moods, Situations)

What I Will Pay More Attention To: (Behaviors/Actions)

How Did I Do Today?

☐ **Brilliant**   ☐ **Really Well** ☐ **Just Okay**
☐ **I'll Focus On Doing Better Tomorrow**

"Take it a day at a time."

Daily Planner

Date: Weight:

Meals	What & How Much?	How was it prepared?	Where did you get your food?	Where did you eat?	Who did you eat with?
Breakfast					
Snack					
Lunch					

Snack

Dinner

Dessert/
Snack

Keepin' Hydrated!
8 x 8 ounces of water each day.

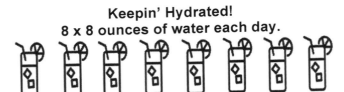

Exercise Today (Time & Type of Workouts)

What's Your Mood: Happy, quiet, sad, hopeful, bored, exhausted, lonely, peaceful, tired, stressed, joyful, calm?   **Make a note:**

What's My Day Been Like? Any Triggers? (Times, People, Moods, Situations)

What I Will Pay More Attention To: (Behaviors/Actions)

How Did I Do Today?

☐ **Brilliant**   ☐ **Really Well** ☐ **Just Okay**
☐ **I'll Focus On Doing Better Tomorrow**

"Pay attention to your thoughts. Are they kind ones?"

Daily Planner

Date: Weight:

Meals	What & How Much?	How was it prepared?	Where did you get your food?	Where did you eat?	Who did you eat with?
Breakfast					
Snack					
Lunch					

Snack

Dinner

**Dessert/
Snack**

Keepin' Hydrated!
8 x 8 ounces of water each day.

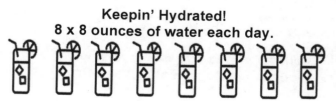

Exercise Today (Time & Type of Workouts)

What's Your Mood: Happy, quiet, sad, hopeful, bored, exhausted, lonely, peaceful, tired, stressed, joyful, calm? **Make a note:**

What's My Day Been Like? Any Triggers? (Times, People, Moods, Situations)

What I Will Pay More Attention To: (Behaviors/Actions)

How Did I Do Today?

☐ **Brilliant** ☐ **Really Well** ☐ **Just Okay**
☐ **I'll Focus On Doing Better Tomorrow**

"Every accomplishment starts with the willingness to try."

Daily Planner

Date: Weight:

Meals	What & How Much?	How was it prepared?	Where did you get your food?	Where did you eat?	Who did you eat with?
Breakfast					
Snack					
Lunch					

Snack

Dinner

**Dessert/
Snack**

Keepin' Hydrated!
8 x 8 ounces of water each day.

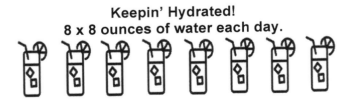

Exercise Today (Time & Type of Workouts)

What's Your Mood: Happy, quiet, sad, hopeful, bored, exhausted, lonely, peaceful, tired, stressed, joyful, calm? **Make a note:**

What's My Day Been Like? Any Triggers? (Times, People, Moods, Situations)

What I Will Pay More Attention To: (Behaviors/Actions)

How Did I Do Today?

☐ **Brilliant**   ☐ **Really Well** ☐ **Just Okay**
☐ **I'll Focus On Doing Better Tomorrow**

"Look in the mirror and see a miracle, because you are."

Daily Planner

Date: Weight:

Meals	What & How Much?	How was it prepared?	Where did you get your food?	Where did you eat?	Who did you eat with?
Breakfast					
Snack					
Lunch					

Snack

Dinner

**Dessert/
Snack**

Keepin' Hydrated!
8 x 8 ounces of water each day.

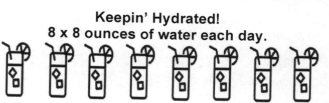

Exercise Today (Time & Type of Workouts)

What's Your Mood: Happy, quiet, sad, hopeful, bored, exhausted, lonely, peaceful, tired, stressed, joyful, calm? Make a note:

What's My Day Been Like? Any Triggers? (Times, People, Moods, Situations)

What I Will Pay More Attention To: (Behaviors/Actions)

How Did I Do Today?

☐ **Brilliant**   ☐ **Really Well** ☐ **Just Okay**
☐ **I'll Focus On Doing Better Tomorrow**

"Every accomplishment starts with the willingness to try."

Daily Planner

Date: Weight:

Meals	What & How Much?	How was it prepared?	Where did you get your food?	Where did you eat?	Who did you eat with?
Breakfast					
Snack					
Lunch					

Snack

Dinner

**Dessert/
Snack**

Keepin' Hydrated!
8 x 8 ounces of water each day.

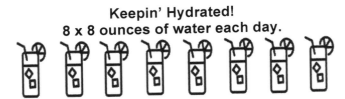

Exercise Today (Time & Type of Workouts)

What's Your Mood: Happy, quiet, sad, hopeful, bored, exhausted, lonely, peaceful, tired, stressed, joyful, calm? **Make a note:**

What's My Day Been Like? Any Triggers? (Times, People, Moods, Situations)

What I Will Pay More Attention To: (Behaviors/Actions)

How Did I Do Today?

□ **Brilliant** □ **Really Well** □ **Just Okay**
□ **I'll Focus On Doing Better Tomorrow**

"Expect and accept that you are going to be successful."

Daily Planner

Date: Weight:

Meals	What & How Much?	How was it prepared?	Where did you get your food?	Where did you eat?	Who did you eat with?
Breakfast					
Snack					
Lunch					

Snack

Dinner

**Dessert/
Snack**

Keepin' Hydrated!
8 x 8 ounces of water each day.

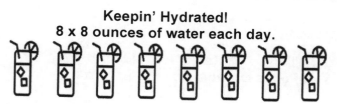

Exercise Today (Time & Type of Workouts)

What's Your Mood: Happy, quiet, sad, hopeful, bored, exhausted, lonely, peaceful, tired, stressed, joyful, calm?   **Make a note:**

What's My Day Been Like? Any Triggers? (Times, People, Moods, Situations)

What I Will Pay More Attention To: (Behaviors/Actions)

How Did I Do Today?

☐ **Brilliant**   ☐ **Really Well** ☐ **Just Okay**
☐ **I'll Focus On Doing Better Tomorrow**

"The world is a better place with you in it."

Daily Planner

Date: Weight:

Meals	What & How Much?	How was it prepared?	Where did you get your food?	Where did you eat?	Who did you eat with?
Breakfast					
Snack					
Lunch					

Snack

Dinner

**Dessert/
Snack**

Keepin' Hydrated!
8 x 8 ounces of water each day.

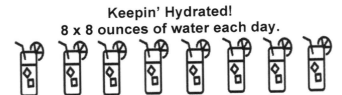

Exercise Today (Time & Type of Workouts)

What's Your Mood: Happy, quiet, sad, hopeful, bored, exhausted, lonely, peaceful, tired, stressed, joyful, calm?   **Make a note:**

What's My Day Been Like? Any Triggers? (Times, People, Moods, Situations)

What I Will Pay More Attention To: (Behaviors/Actions)

How Did I Do Today?

☐ **Brilliant**   ☐ **Really Well** ☐ **Just Okay**
☐ **I'll Focus On Doing Better Tomorrow**

"Small steps equal big changes."

Daily Planner

Date: Weight:

Meals	What & How Much?	How was it prepared?	Where did you get your food?	Where did you eat?	Who did you eat with?
Breakfast					
Snack					
Lunch					

Snack

Dinner

**Dessert/
Snack**

Keepin' Hydrated!
8 x 8 ounces of water each day.

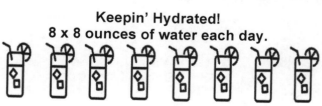

Exercise Today (Time & Type of Workouts)

What's Your Mood: Happy, quiet, sad, hopeful, bored, exhausted, lonely, peaceful, tired, stressed, joyful, calm?   **Make a note:**

What's My Day Been Like? Any Triggers? (Times, People, Moods, Situations)

What I Will Pay More Attention To: (Behaviors/Actions)

How Did I Do Today?

☐ **Brilliant**   ☐ **Really Well** ☐ **Just Okay**
☐ **I'll Focus On Doing Better Tomorrow**

"Be kind to yourself as well as others."

Daily Planner

Date: Weight:

Meals	What & How Much?	How was it prepared?	Where did you get your food?	Where did you eat?	Who did you eat with?
Breakfast					
Snack					
Lunch					

Snack

Dinner

**Dessert/
Snack**

Keepin' Hydrated!
8 x 8 ounces of water each day.

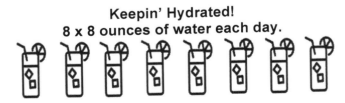

Exercise Today (Time & Type of Workouts)

What's Your Mood: Happy, quiet, sad, hopeful, bored, exhausted, lonely, peaceful, tired, stressed, joyful, calm?   **Make a note:**

What's My Day Been Like? Any Triggers? (Times, People, Moods, Situations)

What I Will Pay More Attention To: (Behaviors/Actions)

How Did I Do Today?

☐ **Brilliant**   ☐ **Really Well** ☐ **Just Okay**
☐ **I'll Focus On Doing Better Tomorrow**

"Every day is a new beginning."

Daily Planner

Date: Weight:

Meals	What & How Much?	How was it prepared?	Where did you get your food?	Where did you eat?	Who did you eat with?
Breakfast					
Snack					
Lunch					

Snack

Dinner

**Dessert/
Snack**

Keepin' Hydrated!
8 x 8 ounces of water each day.

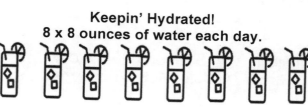

Exercise Today (Time & Type of Workouts)

What's Your Mood: Happy, quiet, sad, hopeful, bored, exhausted, lonely, peaceful, tired, stressed, joyful, calm? **Make a note:**

What's My Day Been Like? Any Triggers? (Times, People, Moods, Situations)

What I Will Pay More Attention To: (Behaviors/Actions)

How Did I Do Today?

☐ **Brilliant** ☐ **Really Well** ☐ **Just Okay**
☐ **I'll Focus On Doing Better Tomorrow**

"You are going great!"

Daily Planner

Date: Weight:

Meals	What & How Much?	How was it prepared?	Where did you get your food?	Where did you eat?	Who did you eat with?
Breakfast					
Snack					
Lunch					

Snack

Dinner

**Dessert/
Snack**

Keepin' Hydrated!
8 x 8 ounces of water each day.

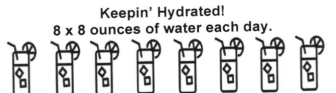

Exercise Today (Time & Type of Workouts)

What's Your Mood: Happy, quiet, sad, hopeful, bored, exhausted, lonely, peaceful, tired, stressed, joyful, calm?   **Make a note:**

What's My Day Been Like? Any Triggers? (Times, People, Moods, Situations)

What I Will Pay More Attention To: (Behaviors/Actions)

How Did I Do Today?

☐ **Brilliant**   ☐ **Really Well** ☐ **Just Okay**
☐ **I'll Focus On Doing Better Tomorrow**

"Every accomplishment starts with the willingness to try."

Daily Planner

Date: Weight:

Meals	What & How Much?	How was it prepared?	Where did you get your food?	Where did you eat?	Who did you eat with?
Breakfast					
Snack					
Lunch					

Snack

Dinner

**Dessert/
Snack**

Keepin' Hydrated!
8 x 8 ounces of water each day.

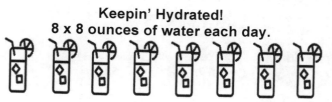

Exercise Today (Time & Type of Workouts)

What's Your Mood: Happy, quiet, sad, hopeful, bored, exhausted, lonely, peaceful, tired, stressed, joyful, calm?   **Make a note:**

What's My Day Been Like? Any Triggers? (Times, People, Moods, Situations)

What I Will Pay More Attention To: (Behaviors/Actions)

How Did I Do Today?

☐ **Brilliant**   ☐ **Really Well** ☐ **Just Okay**
☐ **I'll Focus On Doing Better Tomorrow**

"Just taking action is an accomplishment. Savor it"

Daily Planner

Date: Weight:

Meals	What & How Much?	How was it prepared?	Where did you get your food?	Where did you eat?	Who did you eat with?
Breakfast					
Snack					
Lunch					

Snack

Dinner

**Dessert/
Snack**

Keepin' Hydrated!
8 x 8 ounces of water each day.

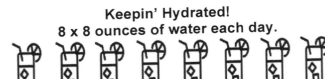

Exercise Today (Time & Type of Workouts)

What's Your Mood: Happy, quiet, sad, hopeful, bored, exhausted, lonely, peaceful, tired, stressed, joyful, calm? **Make a note:**

What's My Day Been Like? Any Triggers? (Times, People, Moods, Situations)

What I Will Pay More Attention To: (Behaviors/Actions)

How Did I Do Today?

☐ **Brilliant**   ☐ **Really Well** ☐ **Just Okay**
☐ **I'll Focus On Doing Better Tomorrow**

"Take it a day at a time."

Daily Planner

Date: Weight:

Meals	What & How Much?	How was it prepared?	Where did you get your food?	Where did you eat?	Who did you eat with?
Breakfast					
Snack					
Lunch					

Snack

Dinner

**Dessert/
Snack**

Keepin' Hydrated!
8 x 8 ounces of water each day.

Exercise Today (Time & Type of Workouts)

What's Your Mood: Happy, quiet, sad, hopeful, bored, exhausted, lonely, peaceful, tired, stressed, joyful, calm? **Make a note:**

What's My Day Been Like? Any Triggers? (Times, People, Moods, Situations)

What I Will Pay More Attention To: (Behaviors/Actions)

How Did I Do Today?

☐ **Brilliant**   ☐ **Really Well** ☐ **Just Okay**
☐ **I'll Focus On Doing Better Tomorrow**

"Every accomplishment starts with the willingness to try."

Daily Planner

Date: Weight:

Meals	What & How Much?	How was it prepared?	Where did you get your food?	Where did you eat?	Who did you eat with?
Breakfast					
Snack					
Lunch					

Snack

Dinner

**Dessert/
Snack**

Keepin' Hydrated!
8 x 8 ounces of water each day.

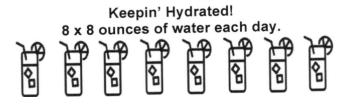

Exercise Today (Time & Type of Workouts)

What's Your Mood: Happy, quiet, sad, hopeful, bored, exhausted, lonely, peaceful, tired, stressed, joyful, calm?   **Make a note:**

What's My Day Been Like? Any Triggers? (Times, People, Moods, Situations)

What I Will Pay More Attention To: (Behaviors/Actions)

How Did I Do Today?

☐ **Brilliant**   ☐ **Really Well** ☐ **Just Okay**
☐ **I'll Focus On Doing Better Tomorrow**

"Every hour is precious. Be mindful of how you spend them."

Daily Planner

Date: Weight:

Meals	What & How Much?	How was it prepared?	Where did you get your food?	Where did you eat?	Who did you eat with?
Breakfast					
Snack					
Lunch					

Snack

Dinner

**Dessert/
Snack**

Keepin' Hydrated!
8 x 8 ounces of water each day.

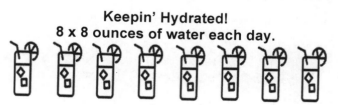

Exercise Today (Time & Type of Workouts)

What's Your Mood: Happy, quiet, sad, hopeful, bored, exhausted, lonely, peaceful, tired, stressed, joyful, calm?   **Make a note:**

What's My Day Been Like? Any Triggers? (Times, People, Moods, Situations)

What I Will Pay More Attention To: (Behaviors/Actions)

How Did I Do Today?

☐ **Brilliant**   ☐ **Really Well** ☐ **Just Okay**
☐ **I'll Focus On Doing Better Tomorrow**

"Every accomplishment starts with the willingness to try."

Daily Planner

Date: Weight:

Meals	What & How Much?	How was it prepared?	Where did you get your food?	Where did you eat?	Who did you eat with?
Breakfast					
Snack					
Lunch					

Snack

Dinner

**Dessert/
Snack**

Keepin' Hydrated!
8 x 8 ounces of water each day.

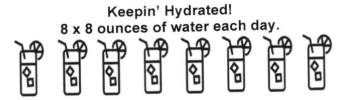

Exercise Today (Time & Type of Workouts)

What's Your Mood: Happy, quiet, sad, hopeful, bored, exhausted, lonely, peaceful, tired, stressed, joyful, calm? Make a note:

What's My Day Been Like? Any Triggers? (Times, People, Moods, Situations)

What I Will Pay More Attention To: (Behaviors/Actions)

How Did I Do Today?

☐ Brilliant   ☐ Really Well ☐ Just Okay
☐ I'll Focus On Doing Better Tomorrow

"Try something new tomorrow."

Daily Planner

Date: Weight:

Meals	What & How Much?	How was it prepared?	Where did you get your food?	Where did you eat?	Who did you eat with?
Breakfast					
Snack					
Lunch					

Snack

Dinner

**Dessert/
Snack**

Keepin' Hydrated!
8 x 8 ounces of water each day.

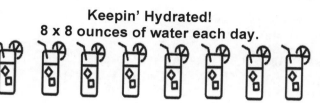

Exercise Today (Time & Type of Workouts)

What's Your Mood: Happy, quiet, sad, hopeful, bored, exhausted, lonely, peaceful, tired, stressed, joyful, calm?   **Make a note:**

What's My Day Been Like? Any Triggers? (Times, People, Moods, Situations)

What I Will Pay More Attention To: (Behaviors/Actions)

How Did I Do Today?

□ **Brilliant**   □ **Really Well** □ **Just Okay**
□ **I'll Focus On Doing Better Tomorrow**

"Look in the mirror and you will see a miracle."

Daily Planner

Date: Weight:

Meals	What & How Much?	How was it prepared?	Where did you get your food?	Where did you eat?	Who did you eat with?
Breakfast					
Snack					
Lunch					

Snack

Dinner

**Dessert/
Snack**

Keepin' Hydrated!
8 x 8 ounces of water each day.

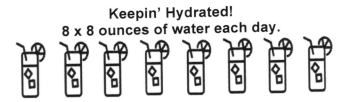

Exercise Today (Time & Type of Workouts)

What's Your Mood: Happy, quiet, sad, hopeful, bored, exhausted, lonely, peaceful, tired, stressed, joyful, calm?   **Make a note:**

What's My Day Been Like? Any Triggers? (Times, People, Moods, Situations)

What I Will Pay More Attention To: (Behaviors/Actions)

How Did I Do Today?

☐ **Brilliant**   ☐ **Really Well** ☐ **Just Okay**
☐ **I'll Focus On Doing Better Tomorrow**

"Listen to your favorite music and feel the joy."

Daily Planner

Date: Weight:

Meals	What & How Much?	How was it prepared?	Where did you get your food?	Where did you eat?	Who did you eat with?
Breakfast					
Snack					
Lunch					

Snack

Dinner

**Dessert/
Snack**

Keepin' Hydrated!
8 x 8 ounces of water each day.

Exercise Today (Time & Type of Workouts)

What's Your Mood: Happy, quiet, sad, hopeful, bored, exhausted, lonely, peaceful, tired, stressed, joyful, calm? **Make a note:**

What's My Day Been Like? Any Triggers? (Times, People, Moods, Situations)

What I Will Pay More Attention To: (Behaviors/Actions)

How Did I Do Today?

☐ **Brilliant**   ☐ **Really Well** ☐ **Just Okay**
☐ **I'll Focus On Doing Better Tomorrow**

"Every accomplishment starts with the willingness to try."

Daily Planner

Date: Weight:

Meals	What & How Much?	How was it prepared?	Where did you get your food?	Where did you eat?	Who did you eat with?
Breakfast					
Snack					
Lunch					

Snack

Dinner

**Dessert/
Snack**

Keepin' Hydrated!
8 x 8 ounces of water each day.

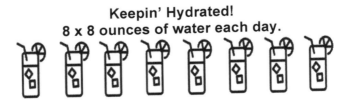

Exercise Today (Time & Type of Workouts)

What's Your Mood: Happy, quiet, sad, hopeful, bored, exhausted, lonely, peaceful, tired, stressed, joyful, calm?   **Make a note:**

What's My Day Been Like? Any Triggers? (Times, People, Moods, Situations)

What I Will Pay More Attention To: (Behaviors/Actions)

How Did I Do Today?

☐ **Brilliant**   ☐ **Really Well** ☐ **Just Okay**
☐ **I'll Focus On Doing Better Tomorrow**

"Every day is a new start."

Daily Planner

Date: Weight:

Meals	What & How Much?	How was it prepared?	Where did you get your food?	Where did you eat?	Who did you eat with?
Breakfast					
Snack					
Lunch					

Snack

Dinner

**Dessert/
Snack**

Keepin' Hydrated!
8 x 8 ounces of water each day.

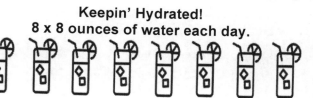

Exercise Today (Time & Type of Workouts)

What's Your Mood: Happy, quiet, sad, hopeful, bored, exhausted, lonely, peaceful, tired, stressed, joyful, calm?   **Make a note:**

What's My Day Been Like? Any Triggers? (Times, People, Moods, Situations)

What I Will Pay More Attention To: (Behaviors/Actions)

How Did I Do Today?

☐ **Brilliant**   ☐ **Really Well** ☐ **Just Okay**
☐ **I'll Focus On Doing Better Tomorrow**

"Every accomplishment starts with the willingness to try."

Daily Planner

Date: Weight:

Meals	What & How Much?	How was it prepared?	Where did you get your food?	Where did you eat?	Who did you eat with?
Breakfast					
Snack					
Lunch					

Snack

Dinner

**Dessert/
Snack**

Keepin' Hydrated!
8 x 8 ounces of water each day.

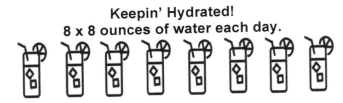

Exercise Today (Time & Type of Workouts)

What's Your Mood: Happy, quiet, sad, hopeful, bored, exhausted, lonely, peaceful, tired, stressed, joyful, calm?   **Make a note:**

What's My Day Been Like? Any Triggers? (Times, People, Moods, Situations)

What I Will Pay More Attention To: (Behaviors/Actions)

How Did I Do Today?

☐ **Brilliant**   ☐ **Really Well** ☐ **Just Okay**
☐ **I'll Focus On Doing Better Tomorrow**

"Good habits are built on small steps."

Daily Planner

Date: Weight:

Meals	What & How Much?	How was it prepared?	Where did you get your food?	Where did you eat?	Who did you eat with?
Breakfast					
Snack					
Lunch					

Snack

Dinner

**Dessert/
Snack**

Keepin' Hydrated!
8 x 8 ounces of water each day.

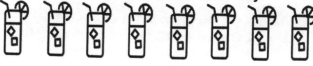

Exercise Today (Time & Type of Workouts)

What's Your Mood: Happy, quiet, sad, hopeful, bored, exhausted, lonely, peaceful, tired, stressed, joyful, calm? **Make a note:**

What's My Day Been Like? Any Triggers? (Times, People, Moods, Situations)

What I Will Pay More Attention To: (Behaviors/Actions)

How Did I Do Today?

☐ **Brilliant**   ☐ **Really Well** ☐ **Just Okay**
☐ **I'll Focus On Doing Better Tomorrow**

"Keep going!"

Daily Planner

Date: Weight:

Meals	What & How Much?	How was it prepared?	Where did you get your food?	Where did you eat?	Who did you eat with?
Breakfast					
Snack					
Lunch					

Snack

Dinner

**Dessert/
Snack**

Keepin' Hydrated!
8 x 8 ounces of water each day.

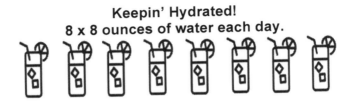

Exercise Today (Time & Type of Workouts)

What's Your Mood: Happy, quiet, sad, hopeful, bored, exhausted, lonely, peaceful, tired, stressed, joyful, calm?   **Make a note:**

What's My Day Been Like? Any Triggers? (Times, People, Moods, Situations)

What I Will Pay More Attention To: (Behaviors/Actions)

How Did I Do Today?

☐ **Brilliant**   ☐ **Really Well** ☐ **Just Okay**
☐ **I'll Focus On Doing Better Tomorrow**

"Every accomplishment starts with the willingness to try."

Daily Planner

Date: Weight:

Meals	What & How Much?	How was it prepared?	Where did you get your food?	Where did you eat?	Who did you eat with?
Breakfast					
Snack					
Lunch					

Snack

Dinner

**Dessert/
Snack**

Keepin' Hydrated!
8 x 8 ounces of water each day.

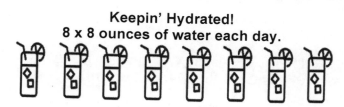

Exercise Today (Time & Type of Workouts)

What's Your Mood: Happy, quiet, sad, hopeful, bored, exhausted, lonely, peaceful, tired, stressed, joyful, calm? Make a note:

What's My Day Been Like? Any Triggers? (Times, People, Moods, Situations)

What I Will Pay More Attention To: (Behaviors/Actions)

How Did I Do Today?

☐ **Brilliant**   ☐ **Really Well** ☐ **Just Okay**
☐ **I'll Focus On Doing Better Tomorrow**

"Expect success and a healthy tomorrow."

Daily Planner

Date: Weight:

Meals	What & How Much?	How was it prepared?	Where did you get your food?	Where did you eat?	Who did you eat with?
Breakfast					
Snack					
Lunch					

Snack

Dinner

**Dessert/
Snack**

Keepin' Hydrated!
8 x 8 ounces of water each day.

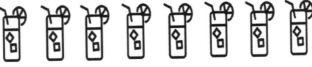

Exercise Today (Time & Type of Workouts)

What's Your Mood: Happy, quiet, sad, hopeful, bored, exhausted, lonely, peaceful, tired, stressed, joyful, calm? Make a note:

What's My Day Been Like? Any Triggers?
(Times, People, Moods, Situations)

What I Will Pay More Attention To:
(Behaviors/Actions)

How Did I Do Today?

☐ **Brilliant**   ☐ **Really Well** ☐ **Just Okay**
☐ **I'll Focus On Doing Better Tomorrow**

"Have a willingness to take action."

Daily Planner

Date: Weight:

Meals	What & How Much?	How was it prepared?	Where did you get your food?	Where did you eat?	Who did you eat with?
Breakfast					
Snack					
Lunch					

Snack

Dinner

**Dessert/
Snack**

Keepin' Hydrated!
8 x 8 ounces of water each day.

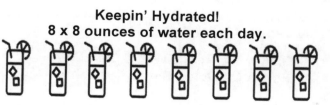

Exercise Today (Time & Type of Workouts)

What's Your Mood: Happy, quiet, sad, hopeful, bored, exhausted, lonely, peaceful, tired, stressed, joyful, calm?   **Make a note:**

What's My Day Been Like? Any Triggers? (Times, People, Moods, Situations)

What I Will Pay More Attention To: (Behaviors/Actions)

How Did I Do Today?

☐ **Brilliant**   ☐ **Really Well** ☐ **Just Okay**
☐ **I'll Focus On Doing Better Tomorrow**

"Every accomplishment starts with the willingness to try."

Daily Planner

Date: Weight:

Meals	What & How Much?	How was it prepared?	Where did you get your food?	Where did you eat?	Who did you eat with?
Breakfast					
Snack					
Lunch					

Snack

Dinner

**Dessert/
Snack**

Keepin' Hydrated!
8 x 8 ounces of water each day.

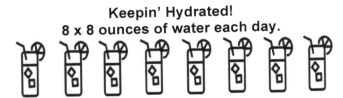

Exercise Today (Time & Type of Workouts)

What's Your Mood: Happy, quiet, sad, hopeful, bored, exhausted, lonely, peaceful, tired, stressed, joyful, calm?   **Make a note:**

What's My Day Been Like? Any Triggers? (Times, People, Moods, Situations)

What I Will Pay More Attention To: (Behaviors/Actions)

How Did I Do Today?

☐ **Brilliant**   ☐ **Really Well** ☐ **Just Okay**
☐ **I'll Focus On Doing Better Tomorrow**

"Be as kind to yourself as you are to others."

Daily Planner

Date: Weight:

Meals	What & How Much?	How was it prepared?	Where did you get your food?	Where did you eat?	Who did you eat with?
Breakfast					
Snack					
Lunch					

Snack

Dinner

**Dessert/
Snack**

Keepin' Hydrated!
8 x 8 ounces of water each day.

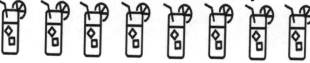

Exercise Today (Time & Type of Workouts)

What's Your Mood: Happy, quiet, sad, hopeful, bored, exhausted, lonely, peaceful, tired, stressed, joyful, calm?   **Make a note:**

What's My Day Been Like? Any Triggers? (Times, People, Moods, Situations)

What I Will Pay More Attention To: (Behaviors/Actions)

How Did I Do Today?

☐ **Brilliant**   ☐ **Really Well** ☐ **Just Okay**
☐ **I'll Focus On Doing Better Tomorrow**

"Every accomplishment starts with the willingness to try."

Daily Planner

Date: Weight:

Meals	What & How Much?	How was it prepared?	Where did you get your food?	Where did you eat?	Who did you eat with?
Breakfast					
Snack					
Lunch					

Snack

Dinner

**Dessert/
Snack**

Keepin' Hydrated!
8 x 8 ounces of water each day.

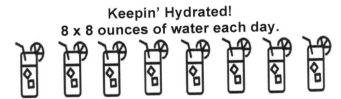

Exercise Today (Time & Type of Workouts)

What's Your Mood: Happy, quiet, sad, hopeful, bored, exhausted, lonely, peaceful, tired, stressed, joyful, calm?   **Make a note:**

What's My Day Been Like? Any Triggers?
(Times, People, Moods, Situations)

What I Will Pay More Attention To:
(Behaviors/Actions)

How Did I Do Today?

☐ **Brilliant**   ☐ **Really Well** ☐ **Just Okay**
☐ **I'll Focus On Doing Better Tomorrow**

"And tomorrow is another opportunity to start again."

Daily Planner

Date: Weight:

Meals	What & How Much?	How was it prepared?	Where did you get your food?	Where did you eat?	Who did you eat with?
Breakfast					
Snack					
Lunch					

Snack

Dinner

**Dessert/
Snack**

Keepin' Hydrated!
8 x 8 ounces of water each day.

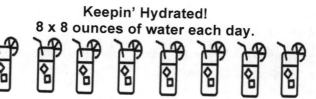

Exercise Today (Time & Type of Workouts)

What's Your Mood: Happy, quiet, sad, hopeful, bored, exhausted, lonely, peaceful, tired, stressed, joyful, calm? Make a note:

What's My Day Been Like? Any Triggers? (Times, People, Moods, Situations)

What I Will Pay More Attention To: (Behaviors/Actions)

How Did I Do Today?

☐ **Brilliant**   ☐ **Really Well** ☐ **Just Okay**
☐ **I'll Focus On Doing Better Tomorrow**

"Every accomplishment starts with the willingness to try."

Daily Planner

Date: Weight:

Meals	What & How Much?	How was it prepared?	Where did you get your food?	Where did you eat?	Who did you eat with?
Breakfast					
Snack					
Lunch					

Snack

Dinner

**Dessert/
Snack**

Keepin' Hydrated!
8 x 8 ounces of water each day.

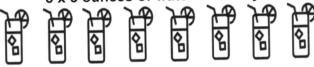

Exercise Today (Time & Type of Workouts)

What's Your Mood: Happy, quiet, sad, hopeful, bored, exhausted, lonely, peaceful, tired, stressed, joyful, calm? **Make a note:**

What's My Day Been Like? Any Triggers? (Times, People, Moods, Situations)

What I Will Pay More Attention To: (Behaviors/Actions)

How Did I Do Today?

☐ **Brilliant** ☐ **Really Well** ☐ **Just Okay**
☐ **I'll Focus On Doing Better Tomorrow**

"Every step equals action. Action is growth."

Daily Planner

Date: Weight:

Meals	What & How Much?	How was it prepared?	Where did you get your food?	Where did you eat?	Who did you eat with?
Breakfast					
Snack					
Lunch					

Snack

Dinner

**Dessert/
Snack**

Keepin' Hydrated!
8 x 8 ounces of water each day.

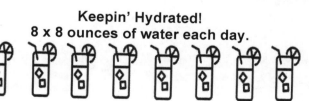

Exercise Today (Time & Type of Workouts)

What's Your Mood: Happy, quiet, sad, hopeful, bored, exhausted, lonely, peaceful, tired, stressed, joyful, calm?   **Make a note:**

What's My Day Been Like? Any Triggers? (Times, People, Moods, Situations)

What I Will Pay More Attention To: (Behaviors/Actions)

How Did I Do Today?

☐ **Brilliant**   ☐ **Really Well** ☐ **Just Okay**
☐ **I'll Focus On Doing Better Tomorrow**

"We all make mistakes. Will you let them stop or motivate you?"

Daily Planner

Date: Weight:

Meals	What & How Much?	How was it prepared?	Where did you get your food?	Where did you eat?	Who did you eat with?
Breakfast					
Snack					
Lunch					

Snack

Dinner

**Dessert/
Snack**

Keepin' Hydrated!
8 x 8 ounces of water each day.

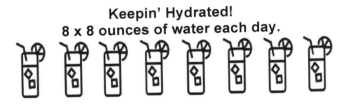

Exercise Today (Time & Type of Workouts)

What's Your Mood: Happy, quiet, sad, hopeful, bored, exhausted, lonely, peaceful, tired, stressed, joyful, calm?   **Make a note:**

What's My Day Been Like? Any Triggers? (Times, People, Moods, Situations)

What I Will Pay More Attention To: (Behaviors/Actions)

How Did I Do Today?

☐ **Brilliant**   ☐ **Really Well** ☐ **Just Okay**
☐ **I'll Focus On Doing Better Tomorrow**

"Every accomplishment starts with the willingness to try."

Daily Planner

Date: Weight:

Meals	What & How Much?	How was it prepared?	Where did you get your food?	Where did you eat?	Who did you eat with?
Breakfast					
Snack					
Lunch					

Snack

Dinner

**Dessert/
Snack**

Keepin' Hydrated!
8 x 8 ounces of water each day.

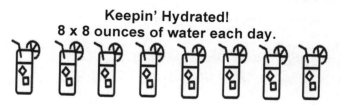

Exercise Today (Time & Type of Workouts)

What's Your Mood: Happy, quiet, sad, hopeful, bored, exhausted, lonely, peaceful, tired, stressed, joyful, calm?   **Make a note:**

What's My Day Been Like? Any Triggers? (Times, People, Moods, Situations)

What I Will Pay More Attention To: (Behaviors/Actions)

How Did I Do Today?

☐ **Brilliant**   ☐ **Really Well** ☐ **Just Okay**
☐ **I'll Focus On Doing Better Tomorrow**

"Every day is a new beginning."

Daily Planner

Date: Weight:

Meals	What & How Much?	How was it prepared?	Where did you get your food?	Where did you eat?	Who did you eat with?
Breakfast					
Snack					
Lunch					

Snack

Dinner

**Dessert/
Snack**

Keepin' Hydrated!
8 x 8 ounces of water each day.

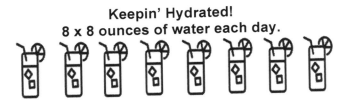

Exercise Today (Time & Type of Workouts)

What's Your Mood: Happy, quiet, sad, hopeful, bored, exhausted, lonely, peaceful, tired, stressed, joyful, calm?   **Make a note:**

What's My Day Been Like? Any Triggers? (Times, People, Moods, Situations)

What I Will Pay More Attention To: (Behaviors/Actions)

How Did I Do Today?

☐ **Brilliant**   ☐ **Really Well** ☐ **Just Okay**
☐ **I'll Focus On Doing Better Tomorrow**

"Keep going!"

Daily Planner

Date: Weight:

Meals	What & How Much?	How was it prepared?	Where did you get your food?	Where did you eat?	Who did you eat with?
Breakfast					
Snack					
Lunch					

Snack

Dinner

**Dessert/
Snack**

Keepin' Hydrated!
8 x 8 ounces of water each day.

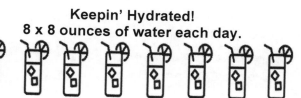

Exercise Today (Time & Type of Workouts)

What's Your Mood: Happy, quiet, sad, hopeful, bored, exhausted, lonely, peaceful, tired, stressed, joyful, calm? **Make a note:**

What's My Day Been Like? Any Triggers? (Times, People, Moods, Situations)

What I Will Pay More Attention To: (Behaviors/Actions)

How Did I Do Today?

☐ **Brilliant**   ☐ **Really Well** ☐ **Just Okay**
☐ **I'll Focus On Doing Better Tomorrow**

"Remember, you've got this."

Daily Planner

Date: Weight:

Meals	What & How Much?	How was it prepared?	Where did you get your food?	Where did you eat?	Who did you eat with?
Breakfast					
Snack					
Lunch					

Snack

Dinner

**Dessert/
Snack**

Keepin' Hydrated!
8 x 8 ounces of water each day.

Exercise Today (Time & Type of Workouts)

What's Your Mood: Happy, quiet, sad, hopeful, bored, exhausted, lonely, peaceful, tired, stressed, joyful, calm?   **Make a note:**

What's My Day Been Like? Any Triggers?
(Times, People, Moods, Situations)

What I Will Pay More Attention To:
(Behaviors/Actions)

How Did I Do Today?

□ **Brilliant**   □ **Really Well** □ **Just Okay**
□ **I'll Focus On Doing Better Tomorrow**

"Be gentle with yourself and expect success."

Daily Planner

Date: Weight:

Meals	What & How Much?	How was it prepared?	Where did you get your food?	Where did you eat?	Who did you eat with?
Breakfast					
Snack					
Lunch					

Snack

Dinner

**Dessert/
Snack**

Keepin' Hydrated!
8 x 8 ounces of water each day.

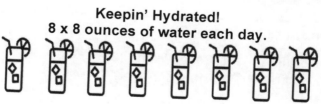

Exercise Today (Time & Type of Workouts)

What's Your Mood: Happy, quiet, sad, hopeful, bored, exhausted, lonely, peaceful, tired, stressed, joyful, calm?   **Make a note:**

What's My Day Been Like? Any Triggers? (Times, People, Moods, Situations)

What I Will Pay More Attention To: (Behaviors/Actions)

How Did I Do Today?

☐ **Brilliant**   ☐ **Really Well** ☐ **Just Okay**
☐ **I'll Focus On Doing Better Tomorrow**

"New healthy habits start with small steps."

Daily Planner

Date: Weight:

Meals	What & How Much?	How was it prepared?	Where did you get your food?	Where did you eat?	Who did you eat with?
Breakfast					
Snack					
Lunch					

Snack

Dinner

**Dessert/
Snack**

Keepin' Hydrated!
8 x 8 ounces of water each day.

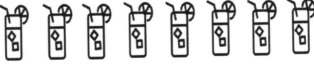

Exercise Today (Time & Type of Workouts)

What's Your Mood: Happy, quiet, sad, hopeful, bored, exhausted, lonely, peaceful, tired, stressed, joyful, calm?   **Make a note:**

What's My Day Been Like? Any Triggers? (Times, People, Moods, Situations)

What I Will Pay More Attention To: (Behaviors/Actions)

How Did I Do Today?

☐ **Brilliant**   ☐ **Really Well** ☐ **Just Okay**
☐ **I'll Focus On Doing Better Tomorrow**

"Every accomplishment starts with the willingness to try."

Daily Planner

Date: Weight:

Meals	What & How Much?	How was it prepared?	Where did you get your food?	Where did you eat?	Who did you eat with?
Breakfast					
Snack					
Lunch					

Snack

Dinner

Dessert/ Snack

Keepin' Hydrated!
8 x 8 ounces of water each day.

Exercise Today (Time & Type of Workouts)

What's Your Mood: Happy, quiet, sad, hopeful, bored, exhausted, lonely, peaceful, tired, stressed, joyful, calm? Make a note:

What's My Day Been Like? Any Triggers? (Times, People, Moods, Situations)

What I Will Pay More Attention To: (Behaviors/Actions)

How Did I Do Today?

☐ **Brilliant** ☐ **Really Well** ☐ **Just Okay**
☐ **I'll Focus On Doing Better Tomorrow**

"Pay attention to how your food tastes."

Daily Planner

Date: Weight:

Meals	What & How Much?	How was it prepared?	Where did you get your food?	Where did you eat?	Who did you eat with?
Breakfast					
Snack					
Lunch					

Snack

Dinner

**Dessert/
Snack**

Keepin' Hydrated!
8 x 8 ounces of water each day.

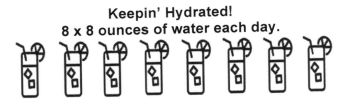

Exercise Today (Time & Type of Workouts)

What's Your Mood: Happy, quiet, sad, hopeful, bored, exhausted, lonely, peaceful, tired, stressed, joyful, calm?   **Make a note:**

What's My Day Been Like? Any Triggers?
(Times, People, Moods, Situations)

What I Will Pay More Attention To:
(Behaviors/Actions)

How Did I Do Today?

☐ **Brilliant**   ☐ **Really Well** ☐ **Just Okay**
☐ **I'll Focus On Doing Better Tomorrow**

"Get out and move, even if it's up a flight of stairs."

Daily Planner

Date: Weight:

Meals	What & How Much?	How was it prepared?	Where did you get your food?	Where did you eat?	Who did you eat with?
Breakfast					
Snack					
Lunch					

Snack

Dinner

**Dessert/
Snack**

Keepin' Hydrated!
8 x 8 ounces of water each day.

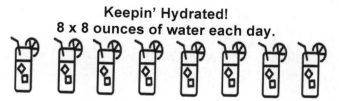

Exercise Today (Time & Type of Workouts)

What's Your Mood: Happy, quiet, sad, hopeful, bored, exhausted, lonely, peaceful, tired, stressed, joyful, calm? **Make a note:**

What's My Day Been Like? Any Triggers? (Times, People, Moods, Situations)

What I Will Pay More Attention To: (Behaviors/Actions)

How Did I Do Today?

□ **Brilliant**   □ **Really Well** □ **Just Okay**
□ **I'll Focus On Doing Better Tomorrow**

"Every accomplishment starts small."

Daily Planner

Date: Weight:

Meals	What & How Much?	How was it prepared?	Where did you get your food?	Where did you eat?	Who did you eat with?
Breakfast					
Snack					
Lunch					

Snack

Dinner

Dessert/
Snack

Keepin' Hydrated!
8 x 8 ounces of water each day.

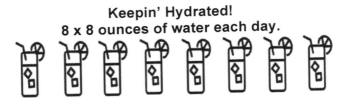

Exercise Today (Time & Type of Workouts)

What's Your Mood: Happy, quiet, sad, hopeful, bored, exhausted, lonely, peaceful, tired, stressed, joyful, calm?   **Make a note:**

What's My Day Been Like? Any Triggers? (Times, People, Moods, Situations)

What I Will Pay More Attention To: (Behaviors/Actions)

How Did I Do Today?

☐ **Brilliant**   ☐ **Really Well** ☐ **Just Okay**
☐ **I'll Focus On Doing Better Tomorrow**

"New healthy habits start with small steps."

Daily Planner

Date: Weight:

Meals	What & How Much?	How was it prepared?	Where did you get your food?	Where did you eat?	Who did you eat with?
Breakfast					
Snack					
Lunch					

Snack

Dinner

**Dessert/
Snack**

Keepin' Hydrated!
8 x 8 ounces of water each day.

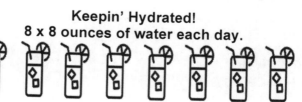

Exercise Today (Time & Type of Workouts)

What's Your Mood: Happy, quiet, sad, hopeful, bored, exhausted, lonely, peaceful, tired, stressed, joyful, calm?   **Make a note:**

What's My Day Been Like? Any Triggers? (Times, People, Moods, Situations)

What I Will Pay More Attention To: (Behaviors/Actions)

How Did I Do Today?

☐ **Brilliant**   ☐ **Really Well** ☐ **Just Okay**
☐ **I'll Focus On Doing Better Tomorrow**

"Every accomplishment starts with the willingness to try."

Daily Planner

Date: Weight:

Meals	What & How Much?	How was it prepared?	Where did you get your food?	Where did you eat?	Who did you eat with?
Breakfast					
Snack					
Lunch					

Snack

Dinner

**Dessert/
Snack**

Keepin' Hydrated!
8 x 8 ounces of water each day.

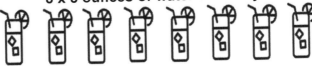

Exercise Today (Time & Type of Workouts)

What's Your Mood: Happy, quiet, sad, hopeful, bored, exhausted, lonely, peaceful, tired, stressed, joyful, calm?   **Make a note:**

What's My Day Been Like? Any Triggers? (Times, People, Moods, Situations)

What I Will Pay More Attention To: (Behaviors/Actions)

How Did I Do Today?

☐ **Brilliant**   ☐ **Really Well** ☐ **Just Okay**
☐ **I'll Focus On Doing Better Tomorrow**

"Pay attention to how your food tastes."

Daily Planner

Date: Weight:

Meals	What & How Much?	How was it prepared?	Where did you get your food?	Where did you eat?	Who did you eat with?
Breakfast					
Snack					
Lunch					

Snack

Dinner

Dessert/ Snack

Keepin' Hydrated!
8 x 8 ounces of water each day.

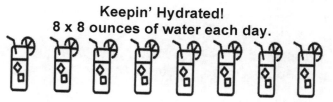

Exercise Today (Time & Type of Workouts)

What's Your Mood: Happy, quiet, sad, hopeful, bored, exhausted, lonely, peaceful, tired, stressed, joyful, calm? Make a note:

What's My Day Been Like? Any Triggers? (Times, People, Moods, Situations)

What I Will Pay More Attention To: (Behaviors/Actions)

How Did I Do Today?

☐ **Brilliant** ☐ **Really Well** ☐ **Just Okay**
☐ **I'll Focus On Doing Better Tomorrow**

"Get out and move, even if it's up a flight of stairs."

Daily Planner

Date: _____   Weight: _____

Meals	What & How Much?	How was it prepared?	Where did you get your food?	Where did you eat?	Who did you eat with?
Breakfast					
Snack					
Lunch					

Snack

Dinner

**Dessert/
Snack**

Keepin' Hydrated!
8 x 8 ounces of water each day.

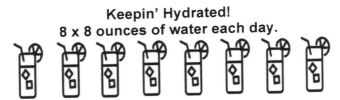

Exercise Today (Time & Type of Workouts)

What's Your Mood: Happy, quiet, sad, hopeful, bored, exhausted, lonely, peaceful, tired, stressed, joyful, calm?   **Make a note:**

What's My Day Been Like? Any Triggers? (Times, People, Moods, Situations)

What I Will Pay More Attention To: (Behaviors/Actions)

How Did I Do Today?

☐ **Brilliant**   ☐ **Really Well** ☐ **Just Okay**
☐ **I'll Focus On Doing Better Tomorrow**

"Every accomplishment starts small."

Daily Planner

Date: Weight:

Meals	What & How Much?	How was it prepared?	Where did you get your food?	Where did you eat?	Who did you eat with?
Breakfast					
Snack					
Lunch					

Snack

Dinner

**Dessert/
Snack**

Keepin' Hydrated!
8 x 8 ounces of water each day.

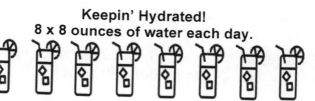

Exercise Today (Time & Type of Workouts)

What's Your Mood: Happy, quiet, sad, hopeful, bored, exhausted, lonely, peaceful, tired, stressed, joyful, calm? **Make a note:**

What's My Day Been Like? Any Triggers? (Times, People, Moods, Situations)

What I Will Pay More Attention To: (Behaviors/Actions)

How Did I Do Today?

□ **Brilliant** □ **Really Well** □ **Just Okay**
□ **I'll Focus On Doing Better Tomorrow**

"Every change can be met with your determination."

Daily Planner

Date: Weight:

Meals	What & How Much?	How was it prepared?	Where did you get your food?	Where did you eat?	Who did you eat with?
Breakfast					
Snack					
Lunch					

Snack

Dinner

Dessert/ Snack

Keepin' Hydrated!
8 x 8 ounces of water each day.

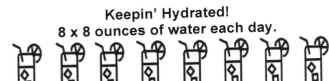

Exercise Today (Time & Type of Workouts)

What's Your Mood: Happy, quiet, sad, hopeful, bored, exhausted, lonely, peaceful, tired, stressed, joyful, calm?   **Make a note:**

What's My Day Been Like? Any Triggers?
(Times, People, Moods, Situations)

What I Will Pay More Attention To:
(Behaviors/Actions)

How Did I Do Today?

☐ **Brilliant**   ☐ **Really Well** ☐ **Just Okay**
☐ **I'll Focus On Doing Better Tomorrow**

"Change is uncomfortable at first, but soon it becomes habit."

Daily Planner

Date: Weight:

Meals	What & How Much?	How was it prepared?	Where did you get your food?	Where did you eat?	Who did you eat with?
Breakfast					
Snack					
Lunch					

Snack

Dinner

**Dessert/
Snack**

Keepin' Hydrated!
8 x 8 ounces of water each day.

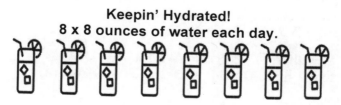

Exercise Today (Time & Type of Workouts)

What's Your Mood: Happy, quiet, sad, hopeful, bored, exhausted, lonely, peaceful, tired, stressed, joyful, calm? **Make a note:**

What's My Day Been Like? Any Triggers? (Times, People, Moods, Situations)

What I Will Pay More Attention To: (Behaviors/Actions)

How Did I Do Today?

□ **Brilliant**   □ **Really Well** □ **Just Okay**
□ **I'll Focus On Doing Better Tomorrow**

"Every accomplishment starts with the willingness to try."

Daily Planner

Date: Weight:

Meals	What & How Much?	How was it prepared?	Where did you get your food?	Where did you eat?	Who did you eat with?
Breakfast					
Snack					
Lunch					

Snack

Dinner

**Dessert/
Snack**

Keepin' Hydrated!
8 x 8 ounces of water each day.

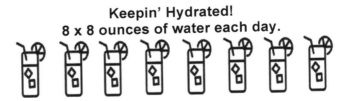

Exercise Today (Time & Type of Workouts)

What's Your Mood: Happy, quiet, sad, hopeful, bored, exhausted, lonely, peaceful, tired, stressed, joyful, calm? **Make a note:**

What's My Day Been Like? Any Triggers?
(Times, People, Moods, Situations)

What I Will Pay More Attention To:
(Behaviors/Actions)

How Did I Do Today?

☐ **Brilliant** ☐ **Really Well** ☐ **Just Okay**
☐ **I'll Focus On Doing Better Tomorrow**

"Take it a day at a time."

Daily Planner

Date: Weight:

Meals	What & How Much?	How was it prepared?	Where did you get your food?	Where did you eat?	Who did you eat with?
Breakfast					
Snack					
Lunch					

Snack

Dinner

**Dessert/
Snack**

Keepin' Hydrated!
8 x 8 ounces of water each day.

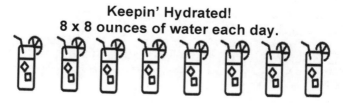

Exercise Today (Time & Type of Workouts)

_____

What's Your Mood: Happy, quiet, sad, hopeful, bored, exhausted, lonely, peaceful, tired, stressed, joyful, calm?   **Make a note:**

_____

What's My Day Been Like? Any Triggers? (Times, People, Moods, Situations)

_____

What I Will Pay More Attention To: (Behaviors/Actions)

_____

How Did I Do Today?

☐ **Brilliant**   ☐ **Really Well** ☐ **Just Okay**
☐ **I'll Focus On Doing Better Tomorrow**

"You've got this!"

Daily Planner

Date: Weight:

Meals	What & How Much?	How was it prepared?	Where did you get your food?	Where did you eat?	Who did you eat with?
Breakfast					
Snack					
Lunch					

Snack

Dinner

**Dessert/
Snack**

Keepin' Hydrated!
8 x 8 ounces of water each day.

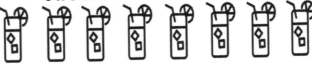

Exercise Today (Time & Type of Workouts)

**What's Your Mood: Happy, quiet, sad, hopeful,
bored, exhausted, lonely, peaceful, tired,
stressed, joyful, calm?**   **Make a note:**

What's My Day Been Like? Any Triggers?
(Times, People, Moods, Situations)

What I Will Pay More Attention To:
(Behaviors/Actions)

How Did I Do Today?

☐ **Brilliant**   ☐ **Really Well** ☐ **Just Okay**
☐ **I'll Focus On Doing Better Tomorrow**

"Small steps equal big changes."

Daily Planner

Date: _____   Weight: _____

Meals	What & How Much?	How was it prepared?	Where did you get your food?	Where did you eat?	Who did you eat with?
Breakfast					
Snack					
Lunch					

Snack

Dinner

**Dessert/
Snack**

Keepin' Hydrated!
8 x 8 ounces of water each day.

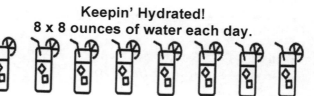

Exercise Today (Time & Type of Workouts)

What's Your Mood: Happy, quiet, sad, hopeful, bored, exhausted, lonely, peaceful, tired, stressed, joyful, calm? **Make a note:**

What's My Day Been Like? Any Triggers? (Times, People, Moods, Situations)

What I Will Pay More Attention To: (Behaviors/Actions)

How Did I Do Today?

☐ **Brilliant**   ☐ **Really Well** ☐ **Just Okay**
☐ **I'll Focus On Doing Better Tomorrow**

"Have a willingness to take action."

Daily Planner

Date: Weight:

Meals	What & How Much?	How was it prepared?	Where did you get your food?	Where did you eat?	Who did you eat with?
Breakfast					
Snack					
Lunch					

Snack

Dinner

**Dessert/
Snack**

Keepin' Hydrated!
8 x 8 ounces of water each day.

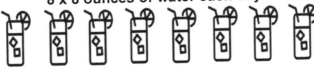

Exercise Today (Time & Type of Workouts)

What's Your Mood: Happy, quiet, sad, hopeful, bored, exhausted, lonely, peaceful, tired, stressed, joyful, calm?　　　　**Make a note:**

What's My Day Been Like? Any Triggers? (Times, People, Moods, Situations)

What I Will Pay More Attention To: (Behaviors/Actions)

How Did I Do Today?

☐ **Brilliant**　　☐ **Really Well** ☐ **Just Okay**
☐ **I'll Focus On Doing Better Tomorrow**

"Congratulations on your new healthy habits."

Daily Planner

Date: Weight:

Meals	What & How Much?	How was it prepared?	Where did you get your food?	Where did you eat?	Who did you eat with?
Breakfast					
Snack					
Lunch					

Snack

Dinner

**Dessert/
Snack**

Keepin' Hydrated!
8 x 8 ounces of water each day.

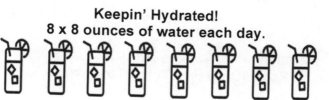

Exercise Today (Time & Type of Workouts)

What's Your Mood: Happy, quiet, sad, hopeful, bored, exhausted, lonely, peaceful, tired, stressed, joyful, calm? **Make a note:**

What's My Day Been Like? Any Triggers? (Times, People, Moods, Situations)

What I Will Pay More Attention To: (Behaviors/Actions)

How Did I Do Today?

☐ **Brilliant**   ☐ **Really Well** ☐ **Just Okay**
☐ **I'll Focus On Doing Better Tomorrow**

"Be as kind to yourself as you are to others."

Daily Planner

Date: Weight:

Meals	What & How Much?	How was it prepared?	Where did you get your food?	Where did you eat?	Who did you eat with?
Breakfast					
Snack					
Lunch					

Snack

Dinner

**Dessert/
Snack**

Keepin' Hydrated!
8 x 8 ounces of water each day.

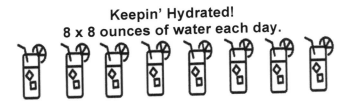

Exercise Today (Time & Type of Workouts)

What's Your Mood: Happy, quiet, sad, hopeful, bored, exhausted, lonely, peaceful, tired, stressed, joyful, calm?   **Make a note:**

What's My Day Been Like? Any Triggers? (Times, People, Moods, Situations)

What I Will Pay More Attention To: (Behaviors/Actions)

How Did I Do Today?

☐ **Brilliant**   ☐ **Really Well** ☐ **Just Okay**
☐ **I'll Focus On Doing Better Tomorrow**

"Every accomplishment starts with the willingness to try."

Daily Planner

Date: Weight:

Meals	What & How Much?	How was it prepared?	Where did you get your food?	Where did you eat?	Who did you eat with?
Breakfast					
Snack					
Lunch					

Snack

Dinner

**Dessert/
Snack**

Keepin' Hydrated!
8 x 8 ounces of water each day.

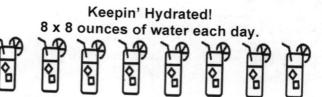

Exercise Today (Time & Type of Workouts)

What's Your Mood: Happy, quiet, sad, hopeful, bored, exhausted, lonely, peaceful, tired, stressed, joyful, calm?   **Make a note:**

What's My Day Been Like? Any Triggers? (Times, People, Moods, Situations)

What I Will Pay More Attention To: (Behaviors/Actions)

How Did I Do Today?

□ **Brilliant**   □ **Really Well** □ **Just Okay**
□ **I'll Focus On Doing Better Tomorrow**

"And tomorrow is another opportunity to start again."

Daily Planner

Date: Weight:

Meals	What & How Much?	How was it prepared?	Where did you get your food?	Where did you eat?	Who did you eat with?
Breakfast					
Snack					
Lunch					

Snack

Dinner

**Dessert/
Snack**

Keepin' Hydrated!
8 x 8 ounces of water each day.

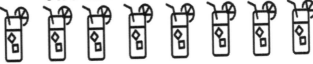

Exercise Today (Time & Type of Workouts)

What's Your Mood: Happy, quiet, sad, hopeful, bored, exhausted, lonely, peaceful, tired, stressed, joyful, calm?   **Make a note:**

What's My Day Been Like? Any Triggers? (Times, People, Moods, Situations)

What I Will Pay More Attention To: (Behaviors/Actions)

How Did I Do Today?

☐ **Brilliant**   ☐ **Really Well** ☐ **Just Okay**
☐ **I'll Focus On Doing Better Tomorrow**

"Every accomplishment starts with the willingness to try."

Daily Planner

Date: Weight:

Meals	What & How Much?	How was it prepared?	Where did you get your food?	Where did you eat?	Who did you eat with?
Breakfast					
Snack					
Lunch					

Snack

Dinner

**Dessert/
Snack**

Keepin' Hydrated!
8 x 8 ounces of water each day.

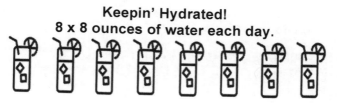

Exercise Today (Time & Type of Workouts)

What's Your Mood: Happy, quiet, sad, hopeful, bored, exhausted, lonely, peaceful, tired, stressed, joyful, calm? **Make a note:**

What's My Day Been Like? Any Triggers? (Times, People, Moods, Situations)

What I Will Pay More Attention To: (Behaviors/Actions)

How Did I Do Today?

☐ **Brilliant** ☐ **Really Well** ☐ **Just Okay**
☐ **I'll Focus On Doing Better Tomorrow**

"You are a miracle."